The Beautiful Skin Workout

ALSO BY MICHELLE COPELAND, M.D., D.M.D.

Change Your Looks, Change Your Life:
Quick Fixes and Cosmetic Surgery Solutions
for Looking Younger, Feeling Healthier,
and Living Better

THE BEAUTIFUL SKIN WORKOUT

Eight Weeks to

the Smoothest, Healthiest Skin

of Your Life

MICHELLE COPELAND, M.D., D.M.D.

with Megan Deem

St. Martin's Griffin

New York

THE BEAUTIFUL SKIN WORKOUT. Copyright © 2007 by Michelle Copeland, M.D., D.M.D. Illustrations copyright © 2007 by Julie Johnson. All rights reserved. Printed in the United States of America. No part of this book may be used or reproduced in any manner whatsoever without written permission except in the case of brief quotations embodied in critical articles or reviews. For information, address St. Martin's Press, 175 Fifth Avenue, New York, N.Y. 10010.

www.stmartins.com

Design by Patrice Sheridan

Library of Congress Cataloging-in-Publication Data

Copeland, Michelle.
    The beautiful skin workout : eight weeks to the smoothest, healthiest skin of your life / Michelle Copeland, with Megan Deem.—1st St. Martin's Griffin ed.
        p. cm.
    ISBN-13: 978-0-312-37077-0
    ISBN-10: 0-312-37077-6
    1. Skin—Care and hygiene.   2. Beauty, Personal.   3. Exercise.
I. Deem, Megan.   II. Title.

RL87.C67   2007
646.7'26—dc22

                                                        2007003242

First Edition: May 2007

10   9   8   7   6   5   4   3   2   1

THIS BOOK IS NOT INTENDED to replace the advice of your physician, whom you may wish to consult before adopting advice concerning diet or exercise, especially if you have health problems.

No doctor can guarantee a particular result for anyone. However, as I explain in detail in the book, I believe that most people can greatly improve the appearance and health of their skin by adopting healthy dietary and other lifestyle changes, and by using a skin-care regimen similar to the one I describe. It is my hope that reading this book will serve as a springboard for improvement in the overall health and appearance of your skin.

The information contained in this book regarding skin care, health, and nutrition is the result of observations I've made in years of practice treating thousands of patients, as well as through the study of relevant scientific literature. Where the literature reflects conflicting opinions, I've expressed my views. You, the reader, should understand that other experts may sometimes disagree.

Finally, the names and identifying characteristics of persons described in the book have been changed to protect their privacy.

Michelle Copeland, M.D., D.M.D.

To Drs. Roderich Walter and Johannes Meienhofer, who opened the world of biochemistry to me when I was a young scientist and instilled an appreciation for the extraordinary value of basic scientific research. To Dr. Donald W. Fawcett, a brilliant cell biologist and teacher who shared the wonder and excitement of life at the cellular level. To Dr. Henry Mankin, a superb surgeon and researcher who gave me the opportunity to investigate connective tissue and cartilage while I was a student at Harvard Medical School, and who showed me how to do many things at the same time.

To my patients, who make it all worthwhile.

To my family, who helps me grow.

Contents

Acknowledgments

This book became a reality with the assistance of many good friends. From the beginning, Delia Marshall and Candy Lee urged me onward. My thanks as well to literary agent Mark Reiter, who believed in the concept, to Diane Reverand, who brought it to St. Martin's Press, and to Jennifer Weis, who guided the project to fruition. Most of all, I am grateful to Megan Deem, who performed the magic of transforming clinical experience into prose.

The Beautiful Skin Workout

The Elbow Test

Touch your elbows. How do they feel? Hard and stiff, like an alligator's hide? Or do they resemble a thick, rigid vintage leather handbag? Perhaps your elbows used to be soft and smooth, but over time the skin is no longer as resilient as it once was. Seriously, go ahead and do it.

I'll tell you why. This book was conceived during dinner at one of New York City's finest steakhouses. I made a wager with my friends. I assured them that I could diagnose the health of their skin right there at the table, just by running my fingers over their elbows. I went around from seat to seat and accurately told each person how often she used body lotion, whether he was a sun worshipper, and the number of lattes she consumed in a day. They were stunned that I could discern so much simply by examining one small patch of skin.

No, I'm not a psychic, nor do I have a supersensory power of touch. I'm a plastic surgeon with a Harvard

Medical School education and a twenty-year affiliation with New York City's Mount Sinai Hospital. I spend most of my waking hours involved with skin, intently examining faces and bodies. I've successfully treated patients with serious burns or large-scale wounds, who assumed their disfigurement was permanent only to discover that the problem could be fixed. I've resculpted, decreased, and created curves and straight lines—all with few to none of the telltale surgical marks.

However, you don't need a medical degree to pull off my dinner party "stunt." Elbows are a litmus test indicating how well you take care of your face and body. If you're fastidious about cleaning, exfoliating, moisturizing, and protecting, chances are your elbows have benefited from this TLC. If you don't like what you see when you look in the mirror, it's because skin reveals all of our secrets. It broadcasts some of those attributes we might prefer to hide: whether we're dining on bacon cheeseburgers, or addicted to tanning beds, or buying our soap in twelve-packs at Costco. Skip the body cream in favor of a pack of Camels, and your elbows will show it minutes and hours later—not years down the road. Skin's immediate response is remarkable. That's the awful news.

The flip side is fantastic. In the same way negative behavior quickly harms skin, appropriate care transforms damaged tissue. That's the underlying premise of this book. There's a simple regimen I call **The Beautiful Skin Workout**, which can not only undo skin injuries but also give your face and body the world-class luminescence you see in fashion magazines and television advertisements.

Does that sound breathless and hyperbolic? Perhaps.

But as you inspect your elbow—even though you're not a doctor—you'll see that the skin falls into one of the following states. Let's count them down according to my nomenclature:

 The absolute worst category is **alligator**. This is cracked, rough, and discolored tissue, akin to an ancient reptile-skin wallet.

 Then there's **leather** skin, which is inflexible and tough with a pebbly texture that comes from years of careless sun exposure.

 Sandpaper is the third designation. Raw and scaly, it's never seen a bottle of moisturizer.

 The fourth, **rubber**, is drapey and dull skin that was once sleek but now resembles a deflated balloon. You can grab it and stretch it with your fingers.

 The fifth class (and we're moving up the quality chain now) is **suede**—passably soft and clear but lacking clarity and silkiness.

 Finally, there's **Creamy.** Creamy skin is flawless, even, and radiant—the perfect combination of glassy and milky, beautiful and healthy. It's skin resembling the proverbial baby's bottom and indicates a life filled with fresh air, vitamins, and organic vegetables. Although surgery can fix a lot, surgical procedures can't create Creamy skin. If you're one of those genetically gifted few who have Creamy complexions without even washing your face, consider yourself extremely lucky. For the vast majority, Creamy has been out of reach from the moment puberty hit.

Until now. We're in the middle of a tremendous revolution in skin care. In 2007, doctors' understanding of skin's cellular structure is so advanced that it's possible to reset its internal clock. Skin has inherent renewal qualities; it's the only organ in which the aging process can actually be *reversed*. Why am I so certain? **The Beautiful Skin Workout** is based on my more than two decades of clinical experience. It's the result of observing what hurts the face and body and what saves them.

I also have a background in biochemistry. I worked in a laboratory for five years, researching peptides and proteins and ways to make cartilage grow, never realizing that collagen regulation would become such an integral part of what I do today. As a result of all those hours hunched over a microscope, when I evaluate skin-care ingredients, I can understand—on a chemical level— whether it's actually possible for them to do what their creators claim. Who would have guessed that diligently figuring out why the sixth carbon atom in a glucose molecule ends up in urine would turn out to be crucial to my livelihood?

To give my patients the best skin possible, I don't limit myself to blades and sutures. I didn't stop researching simply because I left the lab those many years ago. I stay abreast of the latest medical studies, published in peer-reviewed journals, which report the outcomes of trials on everything from lasers to skin-care ingredients. I meet with colleagues from all over the globe to discover the procedures giving them the most success, as well as to share my own findings and observations.

As a result, in my practice, I offer sophisticated noninvasive treatments, such as microdermabrasion, IPL (intense pulsed light), nonablative lasers, and radiofrequency rejuvenation. As we scientists test and retest emerging technologies for skin improvement, we're able to develop new methods for restoring cell function and tissue modulation. I do my own research in the fields of skin care and plastic surgery because soft, supple tissue does more than give you a youthful glow.

Once a person's outward appearance starts to improve, she often feels better about herself overall and may begin making other changes, such as reducing the amount of saturated fat in her diet or putting herself in line for a promotion at the office. I refer to this phenomenon as Cosmetic Wellness. I've seen the positive cause and effect of gorgeous skin enough in my examining room to assure you that it's very real and utterly achievable.

You may cling to the notion that there's always going to be some flaw—a little age spot, a patch of dryness, acne—you have to accept with age. That's like saying we're destined to pack on weight as we get older—despite knowing that sufficient exercise and watching what we eat can help us stay the same size we were in our twenties. To maintain any semblance of physical excellence as the years pass, we must exercise in one way or another. That's so obvious, I almost feel sorry that I made you read the preceding paragraph.

To get skin that's radiant, fresh, and possibly better looking than it was ten or fifteen years ago, we need to put our largest organ on a "workout" routine. We must treat it with the same avid purpose with which we pursue weight loss, muscular strength, or cardiovascular health. In this case, that method is **The Beautiful Skin Workout**. It's a radical idea—we have the power to erase 90 percent of our skin flaws in eight weeks by following this plan—but it's not an empty promise.

I can make this guarantee for two reasons. The first, as I said, is that skin regenerates. Every twenty-eight days, new cells rise to the surface. If you're nice to your skin (rather than insult it), the tissue responds in kind. Second, the body adapts as we continue to challenge it. We've all seen positive results in a matter of days from running on the treadmill or lifting weights. Knowing the skin as intimately as I do, I can assure you that its behavior is no different. If you adopt **The Beautiful Skin Workout**, your face and body's appearance will convert from alligator to Creamy in eight weeks. Period.

It goes without saying that I religiously adhere to my own program. I'm convinced it's effective because people from all over the globe book appointments at my thriving private practice on Manhattan's Fifth Avenue, across the street from the Metropolitan Museum of Art. Among my clientele are some of the world's most well-known, high-profile figures. These are discerning men and women of all ages and nationalities, who demand excellence. If I couldn't make them look their absolute best, I wouldn't have the waiting list I do.

A good family doctor urges her patients to live, exercise, and eat healthily. The more attention you pay to your face and body now, the better they'll be in the years to come. That's why a big part of **The Beautiful Skin Workout** simply advises you to cease doing negative things, just like a personal trainer will tell you to quit smoking or cut out junk food. The other part of my plan utilizes the most recent skin-care advancements to stimulate cell function externally.

As you'll see from my patients' first-person testimonies, obtaining Creamy skin is simple and inexpensive. Once you ascertain your baseline skin quality using the Elbow Test, you'll be able to monitor your improvement during the ensuing weeks. Are you ready to get started on your path to perfection? You've made an important first step just by picking up this book. Now I'm going to guide you the rest of the way with my easy-to-follow, easy-to-understand **Beautiful Skin Workout**. It will work for you, no matter what your age, race, or skin's appearance at this very moment. With a little dedication, your face and body can soon reveal the only truth that matters: how young and vital you *feel*.

Chapter 1

The Beautiful Skin Workout

Today, money is no barrier to some people's quest for great skin. They're willing to pay thousands of dollars to ensure that it looks flawless. They want their skin tightened, taut, dewy, and fresh—courtesy either of the latest miracle cream or a quick trip to the doctor's office. In many ways, they're taken advantage of by a beauty industry that preys on these naked desires. Creamy skin doesn't require a hundred different items specifically tailored for each separate inch of the face or an elaborate application ritual timed to the lunar cycle. All it takes is an educated consumer who's faithful to **The Beautiful Skin Workout** and willing to adopt behaviors that are not just good for skin but contribute to overall health as well. Pretty simple, no?

GUIDING FORCE

With my help, you'll be able to sort through the advice you see on television and in print and discover what's scientifically sound and what's hype. I don't know anyone who doesn't want luminous, healthy skin, the kind that's so soft and unblemished that others compliment it while they seethe with envy. You never hear a person say that she'd prefer to appear wrinkly, with cracked, parched heels and elbows and skin the texture of a gravel path. As much as fashions and tastes change over the years, there is one constant: Clear, smooth, radiant skin is always considered attractive. And this holds true whether you are most comfortable in a pair of Birkenstocks, drinking a mug of steaming herbal tea, or the type of shopper who preorders her seasonal wardrobe immediately after the fall and spring runway shows. I've treated both kinds and everyone in between. An enviable complexion and fantastic body skin, unlike a Chanel haute couture ball gown, are available to everyone and aren't nearly as expensive.

VANITY, THY NAME IS NOT WOMAN

My obsession with Creamy skin isn't just a question of conceit. Incisions in healthy, well-hydrated skin heal faster than those made in alligatorlike tissue. When I see a potential face-lift patient with a leathery complexion, I know that her skin will take longer to recover from surgery. Even if you haven't had surgery, you've likely noticed the difference skin quality can have on another grooming ritual—shaving.

When your legs or face are dry and flaky, they usually become red and irritated after you go over them with a razor. Conversely, the only trace a blade leaves behind on skin that's in good shape is a smooth, hairless area. Proper skin care even speeds the healing process for those who've undergone a rhinoplasty or a face-lift. I always put my patients on a postsurgery version of **The Beautiful Skin Workout**. Oftentimes they come back to me in two or three weeks and say that they've noticed the texture and tone of their skin improving. With this book, I intend to help you achieve the same radiant skin that even my most skeptical patients now see reflected each time they look in the mirror.

FACT VERSUS FICTION

You have to be able to differentiate the hot air from what has proven science supporting its promises. It may seem like a no-brainer now, but when I started out, I was one of the few in my field talking to my patients about skin care. It was hard for me to get them on a consistent, effective routine. They seemed to think that they could ignore their face and body for months, even years, then come to my office and have me solve all their problems at once with surgery. I would have to beg them to start tending to their skin before they scheduled time in the OR. Simultaneously, I was very frustrated by the number of ineffective products on the market and by the amount of money I saw men and women spending on pseudoscience-based creams that made their skin worse. I figured I'd combine my biochemistry background with my deep knowledge of skin to create my own line. It was the only way I could ensure that the same care and attention I gave patients in my office continued daily at home.

Although the phrase "first do no harm" actually isn't in the Hippocratic Oath that all new doctors swear to uphold, it's still a guiding tenet by which most of us practice and minister to our patients. What that means for you is that I'm not going to suggest any products or treatments that haven't been thoroughly tested and evaluated for

BAD MEDICINE

The following material is drawn from recent advertisements and trustworthy sources such as beauty columns. However, none of it is going to give you glowing, Creamy skin.

Moisturize with mineral oil.

Overdose on topical creams such as retinoids, hydrocortisones, and acids.

Scrub with a washcloth.

Shower twice a day in hot water.

Use magnets.

Use skin polishes made of natural walnut shell or apricot kernels.

Wash with Evian or other varieties of expensive, bottled water.

While cleansing with Evian will affect only the amount of money in your wallet, the rest of these "tips" will retard your skin's progress on the path to health and beauty.

safety and efficacy. **The Beautiful Skin Workout** is not about pushing the latest fads; it's a long-tested program that delivers exactly what I say it will. My chemistry training ensures that I understand the formulation of ingredients and how one will interact with another. It doesn't do any good to load your serum with all the latest and greatest technology has to offer if it turns out that combining two ingredients in one solution negates the effects of both.

MIXED MESSAGES

Every day we're bombarded with news on scientific and technological breakthroughs in the skin-care field. The list of powerful antiagers continually swells, with new ones being developed around-the-clock. It's even hard for a doctor like myself to stay current. The rapid progress of research also ensures that magazines and Web sites have an ever-ready supply of recommendations for their readers. This deluge of information can lead to conflicting reports. For example, how do you know which skin-care serum to apply first—your antioxidant or your lightener—when one expert tells you to smooth them on at different times of the day, another suggests waiting fifteen minutes between each treatment layer you apply, and a third says that it doesn't matter at all?

The answer: One of the key elements of **The Beautiful Skin Workout** is learning to think about your skin and what it needs—not blindly following prescribed rules. But since you're just beginning, I'll give you the solution to the layering question. In this instance, it's the antioxidant first, then the lightener, because the antioxidant helps the pigment reducer react faster.

THINKING TOP TO BOTTOM, INSIDE AND OUT

Achieving skin that could star in a beauty advertisement requires a twofold approach. Think about the way you treat your car. You wash and buff its exterior, but you also look under the hood, checking the oil regularly and making sure that the engine is running at its optimal level. This type of routine maintenance means that your automobile not only looks great as you're passing others on the highway but also that you have the horsepower to muscle around those slow-moving trucks. And the chance of you needing to take your car into the shop for an unexpected, major overhaul is remote.

You need to consider your skin in the same manner you do your automobile. Skin is composed of two layers: the *epidermis* (the part you see) and the *dermis* underneath with connective tissue linking the two. Collagen, elastin, and hyaluronic acid (essentially the three main components of youthful, firm tissue) are generated in the dermis. Everything from sun and pollution to a stressful day at the office can lead to the breakdown of these complexion factors. There are ways to build them back up, of course, but as with anything, it's easier to prevent a problem than react to it after it's happened. By guarding against the depletion of collagen, elastin, and hyaluronic acid, you won't have as far to go to reach your dream skin.

I'll get into these safety measures in more depth in Chapters 2 and 3, but for now, remember—these three are the good guys. You want them around, like the party guests who bring you champagne and then stay to help you clean up after everyone else has gone home.

MANUFACTURING PLANT

As the dermis cranks out new cells, it pushes the layers of existing cells higher and higher. These become the epidermis and, eventually, the *stratum corneum*, the uppermost layer of tissue, which—in healthy skin—sheds evenly and invisibly. Blood flow feeds the dermis, meaning that the foods you eat have a direct effect on the job the dermis is able to do in creating firm, plump, complexion-enhancing skin fibers. To return to the car analogy, you can put any kind of gas in your sedan and it will run, but you won't have to worry about pings and knocks if you fill the tank with superpremium unleaded. By this point in your life, you know the kinds of foods you should be eating and the types you should stay away from. What you might not be aware of is that the foods you consume affect more than your waistline; they can also improve the appearance of your skin.

BOTTOMS UP

Drinking plenty of water is another skin-care basic. The standard recommendation is six to eight glasses a day. Water not only helps hydrate your skin from the inside,

RIGHT ON

A more detailed food list is included in Chapter 2, but here are some of my general nutritional dos and don'ts:

DO

Choose items rich in omega-3 fatty acids.

Drink green tea.

Eat organic if you can.

Skip calorie-loaded, nutritionally deficient foods and beverages, like soda and beer.

Snack on fresh fruits and berries whenever possible.

Stock your fridge with produce high in vitamins A, C, and E.

Vary your diet among food groups.

DON'T

Buy foods containing dye.

Consume MSG.

Eat fish, which may contain high amounts of mercury, more than twice a week.

Make fat- and cholesterol-rich red meat and eggs a dietary staple.

Fill up on processed items.

Load your shopping cart with canned or frozen meals.

it also flushes out your system, pushing waste and other by-products through your body, sort of like sweeping off your porch. But drinking eight, or even eighteen, glasses of water daily isn't enough to keep your skin moisturized and supple; lotion completes the equation.

HIT THE BRICKS

Regular exercise should become another of your priorities. Fitness experts recommend a minimum of thirty minutes of cardio three times a week and resistance training twice weekly in order to maintain general good health. Getting your blood going and working off some of your anxiety can't help but improve your skin. By reducing your levels of cortisol, the stress hormone, you'll free your body to focus on other tasks, like building your collagen fibers. Some people enjoy sweating profusely on the treadmill because they believe that's how we rid our skin and internal systems of toxic materials. This isn't true. Only your liver processes and excretes toxins; the skin has nothing to do with it. If pushing yourself to your physical limits makes you feel better, though, that will have a positive impact on your face and body.

IT'S ALL ABOUT YOU

The epidermis doesn't receive any nutrients from the body since there's no blood flow there. Like a newborn baby who relies on his mother to feed and take care of him, the epidermis needs you to supply it with the ingredients that will allow it to grow and achieve its optimal potential. The better shape the epidermis is in, the easier it is to see the effects of blood flow to the dermis—the luminous, healthy glow so universally coveted that beauty companies have made millions on skin care and cosmetics that promise to deliver it. By brushing off loose layers of the stratum

ETERNAL VOW

There's a reason I call this a workout. You have to be committed if you want to enjoy a lifetime of Creamy skin. If you abandon a gym routine after eight weeks, you don't expect that you'll keep the improvements you made in muscle tone and aerobic capacity. It's exactly the same thing when you are taking care of your skin. You floss and brush your teeth twice a day (I hope—I'm also trained as a dentist) not only to keep your enamel white, but also to stave off gum disease and tooth decay. Properly tending to your face and body must also become a part of your daily grooming and health-care routine.

corneum, you ensure that whatever you rub into your skin afterward sinks in deeper. Exfoliation also tells the body to generate new, fresh, plump, and healthy skin cells in the dermis to replace what you've just taken away. You don't need those old surface cells—they're not adding any benefit—but their replacements make your skin more radiant and firm.

EYEWITNESS ACCOUNTS

When a researcher publishes a scientific study, her colleagues will often re-create her testing methodology. By getting the same outcome, they're able to verify her results.

I wouldn't dream of suggesting **The Beautiful Skin Workout** to anyone unless I had data demonstrating the program's success. Throughout the following chapters, you will read actual patient testimonies, in their own words, of their experiences following my prescription. These are an opportunity for an aha, that's me moment. I hope that you'll see yourself in at least one example and that it will help you understand your own situation. My patients' routines included my skin-care products. Having put a lot of time and research into my line's formulation, I believe it's the most effective range available. However, you will be able to achieve improvements by following the tenets of **The Beautiful Skin Workout**. Once you learn which ingredients are important to a skin-care regimen and those causing harm, you'll have the knowledge necessary to make better choices in the shopping aisles. Remain faithful to my guidelines, and I promise, in eight weeks, you'll be looking at a fresher, more radiant you.

WORST-CASE SCENARIOS

I often find that people with skin issues fall into one of three general types:

The Overenthusiastic

Some men and women go overboard when they start exercising, pushing their body too hard, too quickly, and end up with injuries that require them to drop their regimen completely. I've seen similar outcomes from people and their skin-care programs. They figure that if it's good to perform a light acid peel once a week, it must be even better to do one every day. Or that if a thin layer of Retin-A will help clear up their acne issues, then a huge glob of the prescription retinoid will wipe out pimples faster and more effectively. These are the patients whom I end up treating for inflamed, flaking skin or, in extreme cases, raw, open sores. You are not going to see results more rapidly if you double or triple the frequency of **The Beautiful Skin Workout** or the strength of the products I recommend. In fact, you might end up hurting yourself and causing a setback on your journey to Creamy skin.

Reality Show

Sean, 60, attorney

I knew about Retin-A. It rejuvenates and constantly stimulates skin, which gets cells to grow. I'd like to appear less affected by age than my peers, and Retin-A seemed the perfect way to ensure younger-looking skin. I applied it every day. My face got irritated and it was sensitive to the sun, but I didn't believe that anything that wasn't a prescription could work as well as Retin-A. Despite the redness, I kept to my daily routine. I was concerned that if I skipped an application, I wouldn't form as many new skin cells.

Dr. Copeland told me to try her AHA Face Cream and her Revitalizing Formula, which contains antioxidants instead of the Retin-A. I had a hard time accepting the notion that another product could deliver the same benefits, even if Retin-A had its downsides. Finally, she convinced me to switch.

I was shocked by what happened. Now my skin is pretty good, and it never gets inflamed. I thought that I'd need to apply the AHA lotion more often because it wasn't a prescription, but twice a day, as Dr. Copeland suggests, does the trick. The experience certainly illustrated for me the principle that more isn't necessarily better.

The Resisters

On the opposite end of the spectrum are those who refuse to update their skin-care products. I can't understand this kind of behavior. We know that medicine and technology have advanced. Why would you stick to a treatment that you picked up fifteen years ago? I've changed the soap that I use to prep and clean my skin before entering the operating room. I'm fairly certain that you've upgraded your television, or at least thought about it, with the advent of plasma and flat screens and high-definition TV. What may have seemed like a cutting-edge TV set when you purchased it in 1997 probably appears quaint and old-fashioned when you evaluate it today. Sure, you're still able to watch your favorite movies and sitcoms on your old television, but the picture will be crisper and the sound clearer if you switch to a newer model.

Skin-care technology has evolved at an even more rapid pace than electronics. Our current understanding of anti-oxidants, peptides, and growth factors couldn't have been predicted a decade ago. Hanging on to the same cleanser and moisturizer you were faithful to as a teenager means denying yourself and your skin the antiaging and general health benefits of all that time researchers have spent over petri dishes.

Reality Show

Christine, 44, communications executive

Ten years ago, my dermatologist recommended a cleanser and a glycolic acid gel that I'd been loyal to ever since, even though my skin wasn't great. I've always had a lot of trouble with my complexion; I've been on Accutane twice. My face was sensitive and prone to breakouts. I didn't want to try any other products, though, because these were what the doctor had told me to use. He was the expert, you know? I followed his suggestions, and my skin didn't improve, but I resigned myself to the belief that this was just the best it could look.

I made an appointment with Dr. Copeland last year. She told me that skin-care science has changed so much over the past decade; I was really shortchanging myself by adhering to my outdated routine. With just a few simple upgrades in what I applied to my skin, I've seen such a huge difference. My face is a lot brighter, and the texture has improved dramatically. I don't know what took me so long!

The Junkies

Anyone who's having a hard time incorporating new skin-care items into his or her morning regimen should make friends with a skin-care junkie. Junkies have all of the latest and greatest, and their pots and jars of antiaging elixirs are practically full because this type of person is always onto the next thing—including ointments never intended for the face. I've had patients who've tried to shrink their undereye bags with a coat of Preparation H! Needless to say, hemorrhoid cream is not an effective option for deflating puffy lids. But it just goes to show, junkies will try anything, if they've heard from at least one person that it works.

You may be Creamy now, but if you continually switch the items going on your face or body, it won't be long before you find yourself in suede territory. It's always better to be on a regular skin-care program. Daily or weekly alternation of your topical serums and lotions is a form of skin abuse. The tissue reacts by becoming irritated or breaking out. All that back-and-forth shocks the skin; it gets revved up because it's not sure what's going to hit it next. You want to establish a pattern that lulls skin into a regular rhythm. It will be able to function better and expend energy on building new collagen and elastin, instead of working to combat the trauma of a third antioxidant cream in as many days. If it's impossible for you to be single-minded, tiptoe into a commitment by testing my suggestions on a part of your body, such as an arm or one side of your face. Once you compare the skin improvement generated from my method versus your own, you'll be ready to enter into a long-term relationship.

I recently had a follow-up visit with a female patient who'd had difficulty with acne. Her complexion, which had always been in flux, now appeared smooth and glowing. She admitted that she'd finally stuck with my recommendations. And she told me that her new office, unlike her previous one, wasn't near a cosmetics superstore.

Reality Show

Alexandra, 35, corporate public relations executive

I'm a shopper. I read every magazine, and I love to try new things. I'd change my face products at least once a week, mostly because I didn't feel that what I was using was working. Occasional pimples were my major problem.

I was extremely frustrated that nothing completely cleared up my skin. Dr. Copeland explained to me that jumping around with my facial care wasn't giving any of the items a chance to do their job. I'd spent so much money on these various creams and lotions that it was hard to follow her advice at first. But as a plastic surgeon, she's seen so many women who behave just like me. She has to know what she's talking about.

I began using her Rewind Reparative Night Serum and an oil-free moisturizer, and my face looks really good. It doesn't break out, it's plumper, and I appear more rested. My makeup goes on better, too, and my foundation lasts all day. I certainly appear a lot younger than thirty-five!

It's still hard not to buy every new "miracle" wash or cream that comes on the market, but my face has a glow that it didn't have before. I don't want to backtrack or mess anything up, so I'm remaining faithful to her program.

IT'S IN YOUR HANDS

In the following chapters, I'll delve more deeply into what you need to look for on the labels of your skin-care selections. You can see great improvements simply by modifying your products. If you've been lathering your complexion with the same soap you use on your arms and legs, try a facial wash followed by a basic lotion. The results are amazing and almost instantaneous. A specially formulated cleanser won't strip delicate facial skin and make it dry and tight. The plainest moisturizer locks in water and temporarily plumps fine lines, to say nothing of how much smoother skin feels to the touch. Regular body hydration helps maintain skin firmness and elasticity, so thighs are less likely to jiggle, and the upper-arm waddle, the bane of sleeveless-top wearers, won't be as prone to develop. If you can expect those sorts of results just by slapping on the most ordinary cream, imagine what you'll look like once you begin applying things with real power behind them.

LAUNCHING PAD

In the end, the genesis of this book comes back to my inherent desire to help people in need. Just as I want to take aside a woman I see waiting for the bus with a complexion resembling an old cowhide purse, I hope I can aid you on your quest for radiant, smooth, clear skin from head to toe. I am supremely confident in my surgical ability when faced with an extremely crooked nose, and I am certain that by adhering to the steps laid out in **The Beautiful Skin Workout**, your skin will look and feel better than it ever has. You've taken the Elbow Test and figured out your skin's state. Now let's get started.

Chapter 2

The Ten Commandments of Creamy Skin

There is one thing that you, and you alone, can do for yourself: Make your skin Creamy. It's something that no plastic surgeon, no matter how well trained, has the power to perform. I'm referring to a face devoid of brown spots and bumps, arms and legs that are supple and flake-free, a chest with smooth texture and minimal lines—skin that's elastic, clear, and lustrous from top to bottom.

While not everyone can come to talk to me about how to look better, all of us can take simple steps to improve skin quality. In some cases, skin damage is too severe to remedy with anything short of a few laser blasts or a session with the microdermabrasion machine. If that's your situation, you will need to make an appointment with a doctor to see significant improvement. But most of you have the power to create your own perfect, Creamy skin. The process begins by thinking about a part of the body that many of us take for granted.

One of the major reasons I am so proud of **The Beautiful Skin Workout** is that nearly anyone can follow it. Healthy skin is just a few weeks away—a few weeks! Not very long when you consider that a year has fifty-two, and you still have many years left to live. When I tell you that any man or woman will see success, I mean this whether you're eighteen years old and struggling with hormone-induced breakouts, twenty-something and starting to notice that your skin looks uneven and rough, turning thirty with a complexion you feel appears dull and lackluster, evaluating new age spots at forty-five, or in your fifties or sixties and realizing that your face is starting to droop. No matter what your age or how you've treated your skin before picking up this guide, you can transform your exterior surface simply by adhering to my recommendations. In a matter of days, you'll begin to have the kind of soft, smooth skin that you'll be touching constantly, skin that will make others jealous and figure that you must be blessed with amazing genes. More important, it will be skin that makes you feel happy, proud, attractive, and healthy. It's possible to look better than you ever have before—without surgery, needles, massive dieting, $1,000 creams (save your money, they're not worth it), or overhauling your entire life.

Reality Show

Joan, 60, college professor

Even at my age, my complexion was prone to blackheads and breakouts. And I had large pores to boot. Despite the excess oil, sections of my face could get dry and coarse. It was truly a case of, "If it's not one thing, it's another." During my first visit with Dr. Copeland, she gave me a list of items to clear out of my bathroom and kitchen: my moisturizer; my toner, which was mostly alcohol; any high-fat foods—and that was just part of it.

The experience was actually a little traumatic because I had favorites that I used every day. Plus, I had spent money on them, and I didn't want to toss them in the trash, but I did. I started consuming more lean meats and fruit and vegetables. One unexpected side effect of this kitchen makeover was that I maintained my weight during a time when most women can put on a few pounds.

My friends commented on how good my skin looked. They all said they wanted what I was using. My skin texture softened, and the fine lines and age spots receded. The overall tone of my face, neck, and upper chest blended together nicely. I'd never applied products below my face. After Dr. Copeland told me to smooth my AHAs [alpha hydroxy acids] and moisturizers everywhere, I noticed that my jawline and the area underneath my neck tightened.

When I see pictures taken years ago, I appear younger now. When you're eating healthy foods and taking care of yourself, you feel better inside, and that makes your outside reverberate with beauty.

WHAT YOU DON'T KNOW CAN HURT YOU

There is almost always a reason people have bad skin, or skin they're not happy with. I'm not going to lie to you:

Some people are simply genetically blessed with beautiful skin, even though they rarely wash their face and don't seem to have heard of SPF. Don't feel bad—these folks are very rare. Others are born holding the short end of the stick when it comes to their skin: a mottled complexion, constant dryness, a tendency toward acne. Again, these cases are hardly the norm. The vast majority of men and women who have unattractive skin possess complexions and bodies that look that way for reasons that have nothing to do with genetics. It's because those people are clinging to bad habits or are subject to certain skin triggers.

GUILTY PARTIES

Allergies

Bad diet

Drinking too much coffee or other caffeinated beverages

Excessive alcohol consumption

Fluctuating hormones (due to medication or natural cycles)

Harsh, temperamental weather conditions

Medication

Not drinking enough water

Pollution

Pore-clogging makeup

Smoking

Stress

Sun exposure

Unsanitary living conditions

Wrong skin-care regimen or none at all

REPETITIVE BEHAVIOR

I'm sure you've fallen victim to at least a few of the offenders in this group. I certainly have. There's simply no way to avoid the weather or pollution, short of barricading yourself inside your home for the rest of your life. We've all had our share of stress, whether it's due to work, family, or other reasons. If your physician has prescribed drugs necessary for your health, you'd never want to discontinue taking them simply to clear up a few pimples. But many of the factors that cause skin to misbehave or look less than ideal are controllable and, to be frank, very basic. Show me a person who munches on Big Macs and washes them down with Jack Daniel's, and I'll show you someone with blackheads, puffy skin, dark circles, and prematurely aging flesh. Before we can work on modifying your behavior, we need to start with a clean slate.

Ask the Doctor: *Will my pillow cause wrinkles?*

If I told you that it could, would you start sleeping standing up? I hope not. Yes, we do see some wrinkling in hospital patients who lie in one position for a period of time, but does that mean that you're destined for a line-covered face? No. You may want to slumber on your back or, if you're a side sleeper, try switching positions every other night. Silk pillowcases provide less friction than cotton ones, so they're another option to consider. And be sure that you wash your face every night. Hitting the sack with a dirty face pressed into a pillow does more damage to skin than any nighttime position.

FIRST STOP: THE BATHROOM

We're going to empty your cabinets. I know this will be tough for some of you, especially those who frequently update their skin-care routine and have a stockpile of products that's fairly substantial. But if you truly want Creamy skin, you must be ruthless. Fill a trashcan with everything that's keeping your skin from its ideal state.

BAR NONE

It's obvious that cakes of detergent soaps are harsh. Detergents are disruptive by nature. I remember one advertisement showing auto mechanics washing their hands with a certain brand of soap. The implication was that if this bar were tough enough to wipe out grease and oil, the dirt on a regular person would be no match for it. But your body is not an engine that needs to be stripped—and neither is your face. The act of saponification, turning cleansing ingredients into bar form, results in a solid that is more drying to skin than its liquid counterparts. This is the case with all solid cleansers—even "beauty bars." The chemical reaction that stabilizes a bar's components also makes it alkaline, but skin functions optimally in a slightly acidic environment. Gels and anything else in a solution aren't as

---

TRASHY REPUTATION

Bars of soap (no matter how moisturizing they claim to be)

Brushes for the back or face

Loofahs

Rubbing alcohol and any toners that contain it as a primary ingredient (save them in case you need to strip the paint off your house)

Sponges

Vaseline and other thick, petrolatum-based items

Washcloths (if you absolutely insist, you can keep one for your body, but definitely not for your face)

---

detergentlike as cakes, so they're a better option for the face and body. That said, there are sections of our body that can use a little drying, such as the underarms and the groin. It's your decision whether or not you wash with a bar in these places.

Ask the Doctor: *What's the deal with surfactants?*

Surfactants are the ingredients that produce foam in liquid products. They're the reason that shampoos and soaps bubble. They're also extremely drying—for hair and skin. I don't believe they are dangerous, as some claim, or that they damage your general health. However, I prefer creamy, nonfoaming cleansers because they don't strip the top layer of oil from the skin.

Reality Show

Karen, 43, attorney

I'd had microdermabrasion sessions in the doctor's office, and I was pleased with the results: smoother skin, fewer fine lines. My one complaint with professionally administered microdermabrasion was the cost. Like anyone, I appreciate a deal. When I saw a handheld machine with an exfoliating disk head advertised for home use, it seemed like a great idea, because I could do it myself and save money. I was going to share it with my daughter. That way, we'd both have great skin—or so I thought. I began using my new device and I broke out almost immediately.

I went to Dr. Copeland in a panic. She said that the tool wasn't hygienic. Its buffing tip was putting dirt back into my skin, causing pimples. Here I thought that the machine was going to give my face a youthful freshness, and it was actually making my complexion worse.

I switched to her Microdermabrasion Formula scrub, which you apply with your hands, then rinse off. My skin is beautiful again. The cream polishes my face like the professional treatments I enjoyed, but I can do it myself. And my complexion is back to being radiant and pimple-free.

THE BRUSH-OFF

Loofahs are the bane of my existence. You never want to break the normal skin barrier, and that is what loofahs do. I have told many patients to lose the loofah, and they flat-out will not do it. The supposed effectiveness of these scrubbers has become so ingrained in some people's consciousness that it's impossible for them to conceive of exfoliating any other way.

I'm not ordering you to throw away your loofah because I want to torture you. It's an issue of cleanliness and abrasion. Think about how warm and steamy your bathroom gets, particularly the area around your shower or tub. As we all know, bacteria and fungus thrive in hot, moist climates. (That's why you have to clean your bathroom tile with mildew remover.) Granted, it takes some time before the microorganisms build up to the point where you must attack them with a chemical spray and a scouring pad, but just because you can't see bacteria doesn't mean it's not there, growing. Even if you launder your washcloth—and loofah—on a regular basis, as soon as you set your exfoliation tool on the ledge of the bathtub, the bacteria jump right back on. If the idea of cleansing yourself with a fungus-covered item isn't disgusting enough, the rough texture of loofahs, brushes, and other coarse scrubbing cloths create tiny, microscopic tears in the tissue. Skin is our body's natural protective blockade. You don't want to compromise it. Instead, your goal should be to do everything possible to strengthen this outside layer. The small abrasions caused by harsh scrubbing aren't visible to the naked eye, but they're plenty big enough for germs, bacteria, and their counterparts to slide right on in and set up shop. The result, as you probably guessed, can be irritation, breakouts, or worse. If that doesn't have you running out of your house right now to leave your loofah by the curb for the trashmen, then I can't be responsible for what happens to your skin.

Ask the Doctor: *If you've outlawed loofahs, sponges, washcloths, and brushes, what do I wash with?*

Your hands. You should always use your clean hands to wash your face—no exception. The tissue is too delicate to be subjected to anything else. Period. End of story. Body skin is a little bit tougher and thicker. Ideally, if you were using a cloth on the areas below the neck, you'd throw it in the washing machine after every time it got wet. Of course, this isn't realistic. Instead, try to change your washcloth as often as you can and keep it away from any cuts or nicks when lathering your body as the bacteria can slow wound healing. Use your hands on these spots instead.

PERFECTLY POLISHED

I've said no to loofahs and brushes for exfoliating arms, legs, and everything in between. Instead, speed cell turnover with a body polish. Scrubs do a great job. For starters, there's already a bactericidal ingredient in these types of products, so you know your selection won't become full of microbes after the first time you open it. Since you're using your clean hands to apply the scrub, everything—germs, bacteria, dead skin—rinses down the drain.

Ask the Doctor: *How can I get rid of a callus?*

Anything that sits around your tub or shower, such as pumice stone, is going to breed bacteria. Disposable emery boards are a much better option for sanding an area on your hand since you can throw them away after each use. When a patient has a finger callus or tiny wart, I actually have her abrade it a little with a file before applying the medicine at home. With a thick foot callus, you're trying to get rid of excess dead tissue in a larger area. The skin on your feet is a little more forgiving since there's so much distance between the hardened top layer and healthy, living tissue. You can get away with a pumice stone. To disinfect it between uses, boil the tool in hot water or douse it with alcohol. You're no longer going to tone your face with that old bottle of rubbing alcohol in your bathroom, so you might as well use it for something.

Dehydrated skin is often callused because it lacks the plump cells that cushion it against shoes. If you massage your feet with a rich alpha hydroxy acid cream once a day, not only will you moisturize your heels and toes, but the lotion will gently exfoliate your skin. This reduces any hard, thick patches and prevents the formation of new ones.

BUMPY RIDE

Dry brushing is frequently touted as a method for reducing or eliminating cellulite. Proponents believe that going over the hips, thighs, and buttocks in upward strokes with a stiff-bristled brush will increase circulation and break up fat deposits. If only that were true. There's no evidence that anything really gets rid of this type of dimpled skin. Dry brushing stimulates blood flow, which may result in some swelling that makes cellulite less noticeable, but that effect is fleeting. Your skin will return to normal in no time. There's also no topical ointment that will permanently erase an area's "cottage cheese" appearance, although we're working on it. Some products contain caffeine, which can cause a little shrinkage and make skin seem smoother, but it won't last. Endermologie also isn't permanent; once you stop the treatments, your dimples will return. I don't consider it a cost-effective option.

But don't give up hope. There are some scientific advances on the horizon that appear promising, including ultrasonic therapy, light laser sessions, and certain forms of massage. In the meantime, by following **The Beautiful Skin Workout**, you'll make those parts of your body firmer, smoother, and more resilient—which goes a long way toward ensuring that cellulite is less noticeable.

RUBBED OUT

Alcohol is a degreaser. Doctors use it to prep patients' skin before surgery, because we want the area we're about to open to be completely dry and free of dirt and germs. You're never going to be giving yourself your own face-lift, so you have no reason to wipe your skin with straight rubbing alcohol. Creamy skin is about achieving harmony. You don't want it to be constantly shiny and grease slicked, but skin with cracks to rival a desert floor is equally unattractive. Finding a place in the middle and achieving Creamy skin means allowing a little of your natural oil to surface.

The effects from overwashing your face or body aren't dissimilar to wiping it down with rubbing alcohol. "Squeaky clean" isn't a good sound after you shampoo your hair, and it's not music to your skin either. It's an audible clue that you've stripped away the good oils, which, as I pointed out, ends up dehydrating skin and hair. Harsh does not equal clean. For example, brushing your teeth with a hard-bristled toothbrush traumatizes tissue and can lead to gum recession. Dentists always tell their patients to choose a soft brush instead. Your skin is tissue just like your gums. Treat it gently.

Ask the Doctor: *Is all alcohol in skin products bad?*

If you scan the ingredients panel of most skin-care items, you'll see some type of alcohol listed. It's a solvent, which means it dissolves other ingredients in a formula. That's necessary to blend products. Rubbing alcohol is denatured alcohol. Manufacturers take ethanol, the alcohol in liquor, and add a poison to it, so that it is undrinkable. All alcohol solvents contain some of the denatured variety, but we want to keep this to a minimum and use those with the least amount of "poison." Ingredients are listed in order of concentration, starting with the most plentiful and working down. Often water is first. If you find alcohol somewhere near the top and such good additives as antioxidants toward the bottom, the item may well be irritating and less effective.

THICK OF THE MATTER

You may have read about high-altitude mountain climbers smearing their feet and cheeks with a layer of Vaseline. Any petrolatum-based ointment works by forming an occlusive layer over the skin—nothing can get in or out. This is a good idea if you're ascending Mount Everest, where the air loses moisture the higher you go, and you want to avoid your nostrils drying out and bleeding. Unless you enjoy dealing with clogged pores and breakouts, especially on the sensitive tissue around the lips, skip the thick goos in your regular, nontrekking life. You might argue that you apply Vaseline only to your chapped lips, but the product can spread, melting with body heat, and fill up the pores outside the lip line. And it contains no beneficial ingredients, other than to lock in the water already present in the cells. Add it to the trash pile.

At this point, you should be looking at a cleaner bathroom shelf and a wastebasket that's getting full. I'll cover what you want to get to refill your medicine cabinet in the next chapter. Right now, we need to head to another room.

NEXT STOP: THE KITCHEN

If you're committed to reaching Creamy skin in the shortest amount of time possible, open your refrigerator. We're all intelligent people. I'm sure you already know the kinds of food that will make you feel healthy and upbeat, and you're aware of the things you shouldn't be putting in your mouth.

GOOD-BYE, OLD FRIENDS

Fried foods

Grain alcohol, such as vodka, whiskey, and rum

Rich, fatty foods, like heavy cheese, ice cream, and fatty cuts
   of meat

Soda, regular and diet

FOOD FOR THOUGHT

You are what you eat, as the saying goes. Doctors are learning more and more about how a healthy diet helps ensure a longer life. We know about bad cholesterol and good cholesterol and the ways they affect our body and our organs. Skin is an outward reflection of the internal situation. There are certain foods, especially those filled with sugar, that stimulate insulin production, which may, in turn, kick-start glandular pumping. Hops, for example, are the main ingredient in beer. They also encourage insulin manufacturing. If you drink soda all day, even diet, you're consuming fluids that don't contain vitamins or have much internal hydration ability. You're just getting a lot of chemicals or sugar or both, and bypassing the chance to fill your body with liquids, which could make your skin look and feel good. It's a missed opportunity.

It's not that what you're eating or drinking directly affects the skin, but it can indirectly cause more trouble than you might imagine. If your bad cholesterol rises, you're going to have a myriad of health problems because you're stuffing yourself with saturated fat. Those clogged

---

GROCERY LIST

This is just a taste of the items that should fill your cart.

Fruit: Berries, grapefruit, grapes, and oranges—all contain antioxidants, vitamin C, and phytochemicals that may reduce the incidence of chronic disease.

Green leafy vegetables: Broccoli, brussels sprouts, and spinach—they're rich in fiber, vitamin A, calcium, and antioxidants.

Herbs and spices: Cumin, rosemary, and thyme—there's no reason your food has to be bland. These three herbs also pack high levels of antioxidants and give a kick to entrées and side dishes.

Meat: Lean proteins, such as chicken (without the skin) and fish, provide protein without high amounts of cholesterol. They're also low in fat. Due to risk of mercury overload, I don't recommend eating fish more than twice a week.

---

blood vessels also result in a decrease in overall circulation, which translates to less nourishment getting to your skin.

Ask the Doctor: *Should I take special supplements to make my skin look its best?*

As I say time and again in this book, so much of what's on the beauty market today is simply hype. Manufacturers want to sell products and make money. They continue to dream up new and different things, which they can convince you that you need. Pills are no substitute for the vitamins and minerals in whole foods. If you adhere to the dietary guidelines I've set out, you will be providing your body with more than enough of the nutrients necessary for achieving Creamy skin.

SALAD DAYS

I'm sure some of you are reading this dietary list and are about ready to give up. I can never have another french fry? My steak days are over? No and no. We have to live, and we have to be sensible. Am I saying that you can't ever drink a cocktail if you want Creamy skin? That's absurd. In the beginning of Chapter 1, I told you that an essential part of my program was for you to learn to think about your skin and its requirements at that moment. What you choose to eat is simply another fact to enter into your mental equations. Alcohol affects the liver and causes dehydration. If you glance in the mirror one morning and think that your face is looking a little crepey and sallow, it's probably not the best idea to compound those issues by doing something that could make your skin even drier and less radiant. On days when your complexion is glowing, snacking on a KFC Extra Crispy chicken breast or meeting friends for after-work martinis isn't instantly going to send your skin from Creamy back to rubber.

Ask the Doctor: *What's the French connection?*

It's the polyphenols. Now we know that in red—and, to some extent, white—wine, the grape seed extract is a very powerful antioxidant. Researchers looked to see why there was less heart disease in certain parts of the world, even though the inhabitants didn't seem to deny themselves much butter, cheese, or other high-fat foods. They discovered that regular glasses of red wine were also part of those people's dietary plan and the polyphenols in the wine seemed to counteract whatever damage the rest of the food was doing. A recent study from the Mount Sinai School of Medicine in New York City found that white wine also has positive implications for heart health. We've since proved that polyphenols benefit the skin, too, increasing its clarity and strengthening the tissue. A glass of wine in the evening might also help erase the stress of your day and that definitely helps your outward appearance.

SECRETS AND LIES

Growing up, we were told that eating deep-fried foods and chocolate would lead to breakouts. Then experts said that this wasn't true. The current food/acne theories continue on this cyclical track. Certainly, consuming a lot of greasy burgers and heaping plates of nachos with extra cheese does stimulate the glands, so they produce more secretions. If you have a natural tendency toward pimples, a diet high in saturated fat will exacerbate it. Conventional wisdom once also linked chocolate to problem skin. Now the thinking is that it may be the caffeine in chocolate that creates inflammation, not the cocoa itself. Even better news for those with a sweet tooth: The polyphenols in dark chocolate could help skin maintain a youthful appearance.

THE TEN COMMANDMENTS OF HEALTHY SKIN

Thanks to our visits to your bathroom and kitchen, we've cleared away some roadblocks on your path to Creamy skin. You are, in essence, a blank page, so let me impress upon you the guiding principles of **The Beautiful Skin Workout**. I'm giving you a complete program to deliver your best skin possible in the shortest amount of time. In some ways, it's like a diet. When you try a new weight-loss plan, you receive a prescribed list of what to eat, how much, and when. If the rules seem overwhelming at first, you might start by only cutting out the midnight snacks. The numbers on the scale will go down, perhaps not as quickly as if you made more reductions in your daily caloric intake, but you will see a change. The most important part of my program is that you stick to it. It won't work otherwise. If you can commit to only a few of my suggestions, that's okay. Just as a dieter who sees that her clothes are fitting better may be inspired to adopt more of the eating recommendations, once you begin to have improvements in your skin, you may decide that you want to speed up the process and incorporate more of **The Beautiful Skin Workout** into your life. However, if you do absolutely nothing but follow these ten rules, I guarantee that your skin will improve.

THE TEN COMMANDMENTS OF HEALTHY SKIN

1. Thou shalt wear sun protection.
2. Thou shalt clean your face at least once a day.
3. Thou shalt not subject yourself to extremes, whether excessive UV exposure, binge drinking and eating, or wildly fluctuating water temperatures.
4. Thou shalt treat your body's skin as well as you do your face.
5. Thou shalt learn how to exfoliate properly and do it religiously.
6. Thou shalt eat a healthy, balanced diet—and drink a lot of water.
7. Thou shalt slather on such antioxidants as vitamins E and C or green tea every day.
8. Thou shalt not be afraid of pigment-reducing creams; use them daily.
9. Thou shalt make antiaging creams and serums your new best friends and apply them at least once a day.
10. Thou shalt not smoke.

Reality Show

Margaret, 64, retired

I'd always taken care of my skin, and I wasn't a sunbather. But I'd never thought about much more than my face. Imagine how upset I was when I began to notice age spots on my hands and a few on my cheeks. And in terms of my body, the skin always felt dry.

One thing that Dr. Copeland brought to my attention was that hands show age just as much as the face does. I started applying her Revitalizing Formula with vitamins C and E and her Pigment Formula to both body parts. What a difference. The dark patches have really faded. I had pretty much quit wearing rings and bracelets because of the way my hands looked. Not wearing jewelry is a sin in Texas, where I live. Now my hands are so much more attractive that I'm wearing everything at once.

I was washing my body with bar soap and slapping on baby oil. I swapped those for her Bath/Shower Gelee and began rubbing her AHA Body Smoothing Lotion under her Body Moisturizing Lotion. My skin is much softer and suppler than it was before. And I don't have any of those bumps you can get on your arms when they're dehydrated.

COMMANDMENT 1: THOU SHALT WEAR SUN PROTECTION

The rate of skin cancer in the United States is increasing. According to the Centers for Disease Control and Prevention, more than one million cases of basal or squamous cell carcinoma are diagnosed each year. Melanoma, the most dangerous form of skin cancer, is also the most common cancer among those twenty-five to twenty-nine years old. Besides encouraging skin cancer formation, sun exposure is one of the major causes of wrinkles. Solar radiation radically alters your cells and DNA. And it triggers the release of free radicals, which weaken skin's collagen and elastin—the very same stuff that people spend tens of thousands of dollars a year injecting back into their faces with varying degrees of success.

There's no excuse for not rubbing an SPF-rich lotion onto exposed skin daily. However, I don't think that you have to be pale to be healthy. I enjoy spending weekends outdoors, which means being in the sun. You can have some color in your skin, but the key word is *some*. The tan, tan look is counterproductive to being healthy. No matter what tanning bed manufacturers claim about the emotional well-being benefits of a few minutes in one of those UV coffins, I strongly advise you to stay away. Constantly irradiating your cells to keep them deeply bronzed increases your chances of developing skin cancer significantly more than a person who applies, and regularly reapplies, an adequate level of SPF throughout the day.

 Ask the Doctor: *What's SPF?*

Sun protection factor (SPF) is a measure of how long a person can stay in the sun before burning. An SPF 30 means thirty times longer than if you went outside with nothing on. It's important to keep in mind that all skins are different. A woman with an Irish heritage and an extremely pale complexion might last only a minute or two before her bare skin turns pink, so an SPF 30 would give her thirty minutes before she needed to reapply, assuming she wasn't jumping in the pool or perspiring. Her Latina friend, on the other hand, could perhaps go two hours or more before her unguarded skin became tender. The same SPF 30 lotion would extend that time even more. SPF measures only a product's ability to block UVB (burning) rays. A cream's power to shield skin from UVA (aging) rays is not currently indicated on a package's label. And UVA rays are the ones that break down the collagen and elastin fibers supporting skin— no matter how much melanin is there naturally or how hard it is for a person to burn. It doesn't matter what your nationality is. If you don't want wrinkles, you need to guard yourself from UVA light.

Ask the Doctor: *Is there a difference between sunblock and sunscreen?*

The active ingredients for both types of UV protection are listed in a separate box on the label, usually near the top of the tube. Sunblocks typically contain zinc oxide or titanium dioxide. Those are physical barriers, which means that they sit on top of the skin and reflect the rays off it. Everyone associates zinc oxide with white-nosed lifeguards, but the mineral is micronized now and invisible when applied. You can find zinc oxide and titanium dioxide in both drug and department store SPF lotions, sprays, and gels.

Sunscreens are chemical UV shields. They sink into tissue. When light hits them, it creates a reaction that neutralizes the radiation. Avobenzone (also called Parsol 1789), Helioplex, and Mexoryl are the three most effective in this category. Again, these ingredients are widely available across a range of price points and SPF formulations.

RAY BANS

I prefer blocks to the screen versions because their zinc and titanium mineral base induces less chafing than chemical formulas. A block's ingredients don't break down in the sun, which is the major complaint about most chemical UV guards. Plus, zinc is a powerful antioxidant that helps in the wound-healing process. If it's in your sun protection, not only will you be guarded from the rays, but any UV-related inflammation will be treated at the same time. Today we should expect sunblocks and sunscreens to contain other ingredients, like antioxidants, that repair and protect simultaneously.

On a regular day, an SPF 30 with UVA protection is enough, but if you're going out under the midday sun or you're planning to spend a lot of time outside, an SPF 20 or 30 is not adequate. You need an SPF 40 or higher. Anything over 40 is problematic, as the FDA doesn't monitor SPFs as strictly above 40. You might not be getting the equivalent increase in effect that you're expecting.

SKIN CANCER ALERT

I said earlier that you can create Creamy skin without ever stepping inside a doctor's office. That is absolutely true. But only a qualified, experienced physician can check your body for the signs of potential skin cancer, like irregularly shaped moles. In addition to monitoring your skin on your own for any changes, which is crucial (you'll pick up a new growth faster than a doctor will because you see your skin daily), you need to schedule an annual full-body exam administered by a physician. You should go more often if you have a family history of skin cancer or if you used to spend every day broiling under the sun. Fall is usually a good time for the appointment as it follows the season in which we typically get our greatest amount of sun exposure all year.

Ask the Doctor: *My skin tone is naturally deep. I don't have to worry about going in the sun, right?*

Melanin is in our skin for a reason: It helps shield the tissue from absorbing too much UV light. But that doesn't give non-Caucasians a free pass for skipping sunblock. Even highly pigmented skin can be damaged by ultraviolet light. Though her complexion may not appear wrinkled, a woman with a deeper complexion can still end up with pigment variation, usually mottled, caused by sun exposure. And skin cancer should be the concern of every man, woman, and child on the planet Earth.

COMMANDMENT 2: THOU SHALT CLEAN YOUR FACE AT LEAST ONCE A DAY

It's essential to wash your face at night, both to remove makeup and to rinse away the dirt and pollution that your skin picked up during the course of your day. This frees the pores from potential clogs and, in my opinion, is just a basic element of good personal hygiene akin to brushing your teeth. You may wonder if you need to lather your face again after you get up, arguing that since you've been asleep in the dark on your clean sheets, your skin hasn't been subjected to loads of grime. **The Beautiful Skin Workout** isn't magic; it's effective only if you stick to it. If a single daily face wash is all you can manage, so be it. I will point out, though, that your body is working—hard—while you sleep.

Our internal repair processes are going full speed ahead once we head off to dreamland. Core temperatures rise during the nightly snooze. That's the reason some people suggest applying antiperspirants before bed. Your nocturnal sweat will kick the antiperspirant into forming the tiny plugs that block sweat production. As a result, your underarms will already be equipped to handle whatever the day brings, instead of reacting, visibly, to the stress when it occurs. These little pore corks will stay in place, even if you

RULES FOR LIVING

Never go to sleep without removing your makeup—the reason is obvious.

Always wash your face after exercising—your pores are extremely vulnerable once your body is heated up and your blood is flowing. The last thing you want seeping into your skin is sweat mixed with dirt from the mat on which you did your sit-ups.

shower the next morning. Reapplying your antiperspirant afterward will provide an additional dose of protection. I like to wash my face and body after I wake up, simply because I know that I was perspiring while I was asleep. But it's up to you.

COMMANDMENT 3: THOU SHALT NOT SUBJECT YOURSELF TO EXTREMES, WHETHER EXCESSIVE UV EXPOSURE, BINGE DRINKING AND EATING, OR WILDLY FLUCTUATING WATER TEMPERATURES

I continually impress upon my patients the need for balance—between work and pleasure activities, wild nights and quiet evenings at home, not caring for their skin and becoming completely consumed by it. When you're always at either end of the spectrum, you burn out or slip into complacency. For optimal function, your body, like your mind, needs to be stimulated and engaged without being driven to distraction. Establishing equilibrium is essential to health and happiness.

It's also a major factor in reaching your goal of Creamy skin. I hope by now I've made crystal clear the reasons why you should avoid crisping in the sun. You've also seen how what you put in your mouth can have a huge effect on the way you look on the outside, to say nothing of the weight you'll gain and health problems you may develop by regularly gorging yourself. Now let's turn to what you're doing when you're in the shower or bathtub.

THE HOT ZONE

We often assume that something isn't really clean unless it's been boiled. It's true that we sterilize surgical instruments in an autoclave, which uses superheated steam to kill bacteria and other microorganisms. But those tools are made of stainless steel; they can withstand that kind of abuse. Your skin is not a scalpel, and it doesn't need to be sterilized. Certain bacteria are actually good for your health. Washing with hot water dehydrates the skin by removing its inherent oils. Scalding your skin causes injury. That thermal effect can actually damage cell tissue, so keep your water temperature at a warm, comfortable level. The cleanser you're lathering onto your face and body will be plenty effective to wash away dirt, excess oil, and germs.

 Ask the Doctor: *Do I have to stay out of the sauna?*

If I'm telling you that excess heat can be a bad thing, what does this mean for saunas and steam baths? I like going in a sauna. Sitting in dry heat or in a steam room is not a bad thing if doing so relaxes you, as reducing your stress level has a positive effect on skin. Daily sauna or steam sessions are not a good idea, though. Neither is using a facial steamer every day at home. Overexposure to heat and steam will lead to dehydration. Again, it's about listening to your skin. People react to high temperatures in different ways. You might be okay going a few times a week. I'd say that staying in a sauna or steam bath for five to ten minutes is fine; twenty-minute stretches are too long.

If you're availing yourself of the facilities at the gym, you need to give yourself a quick rinse before you enter one of those hot boxes. The heat drives the grime and perspiration resulting from your workout into your pores. After you come out of the sauna, cleanse your face and body, as the increased temperature will have made your skin more vulnerable to absorbing anything, such as perspiration, with which it comes in contact. By the same token, it's an excellent time to apply skin-care products to your washed self, as they'll sink into the still-warm tissue.

FAIR WEATHER FRIEND

Shifting climates can also affect skin quality. In an ideal world, we'd all reside in temperate zones with a consistent temperature and humidity. But this is reality. You're not going to move, so you need to be cognizant of the ways your face and body may react simply because of the place that you call home.

Skin is a barrier, but it's also a way to exchange oxygen and fluids with the environment in a process known as transpiration. If you're in an arid climate, you have to drink more water, because you're not going to absorb enough moisture from the air. Forget the sun—humidity alone can alter skin quality. Glands may have to produce more sweat, and that stimulation results in a greater amount of oil.

HARDER TO BREATHE

Pollutants are another factor. They clog both the pores and your lungs. You're not able to oxygenate as well if your lungs aren't clear, so the blood supply to the dermis isn't as robust as it could be. Pollution can also set your skin up for infection or trigger acne. By being aware that these are problems that may crop up, you can learn to anticipate your reaction and plan ways to minimize or eliminate the effects. It may be necessary for you to adjust your cleansing and toning regimen, such as doing it more often. You might also want to increase the amount of antioxidants and vitamins you're applying to your skin, as well as supplement the level of antioxidants and vitamins you're getting through your diet. This will strengthen your body's ability to ward off pollution-related attacks.

COMMANDMENT 4: THOU SHALT TREAT YOUR BODY'S SKIN AS WELL AS YOU DO YOUR FACE

Some women (and men) are totally focused on caring for their faces. They're fastidious, and they do everything right: constantly wear SPF; shade themselves with a large-brim, opaque hat when outdoors; generously apply anti-aging topicals—antioxidants and peptides—and, in short, remain faithful to their skin-care program. They're rewarded with complexions that are radiant, supple, glowing, and firm. These same people who are so careful about tending to their faces often forget that skin doesn't end below the neck. Having healthy, beautiful skin means looking after all of it from hairline to heel.

WHEN TOO MUCH IS JUST TOO MUCH

So many products on the market are about just that: marketing. Do you really need creams and serums that are specific to each section of the body: legs, breasts, upper arms, and more? That's overkill. I don't believe that your body skin requires a million individual items. **The Beautiful Skin Workout** combines balance with practicality. There's no reason to go overboard or load your countertop with hundreds of bottles. Many of the ingredients I'll suggest for your face work equally well on the rest of you, as long as you apply them consistently. Soon you'll have a décolletage firm and free of brown spots, feet that are ready to be exposed in the strappiest of sandals, and a back that's so soft your dance partner won't want to let go. And turning your skin care into a whole-body affair truly will not add much more time to your normal grooming routine.

COMMANDMENT 5: THOU SHALT LEARN HOW TO EXFOLIATE PROPERLY AND DO IT RELIGIOUSLY

Taking off dead skin cells makes the newly exposed tissue fuller and more brilliant. Your body sheds this top layer naturally, but this regeneration process slows as we age, making exfoliation more critical for a woman in her midthirties than one who's twenty-two. You'll get a greater glow if you slough off excess cells with an exfoliant, either physical (one with particles that you rub in, then rinse off) or chemical (a product containing ingredients, such as glycolic or lactic acid, that melt the glue holding wizened cells on the skin's surface). One caveat: I've seen the damage from overzealous do-it-yourself chemical peels. Acids are simultaneously good and bad. They do a wonderful job of freshening a complexion. Improperly formulated, they can cause burns and scars.

Ridding yourself of this keratinized tissue also permits antioxidants, pigment reducers, antiaging serums, and moisturizers to enter skin effortlessly. The act of exfoliation also stimulates the cells below the surface. They react by increasing their production of skin-enhancing collagen and elastin fibers. Its benefits are, therefore, both immediate and long-term. I suggest exfoliating twice daily. Alligator and leather skins, which are thick and tough, won't have a problem with this. Skin types that are already slightly supple, such as

SAFETY ZONE

Acids that are okay for daily use:

Alpha hydroxy
Beta hydroxy
Glycolic
Lactic (mandelic)
Salicylic

suede, should see how their tissue reacts. If it's red, wait a day before exfoliating again. When you notice your skin developing a tolerance, incorporate the exfoliation step into your regular, everyday practice. You can exfoliate every day with a mild acid lotion; scrubs can be harsher and shouldn't be used more than two or three times a week.

HOME IMPROVEMENT

What scare me are the once-a-week DIY chemical peels I see advertised on late-night television. It's shocking. These products are often touted as containing very high concentrations of acid, levels that I consider dangerous. When I do even a light peel in my office, I have to monitor the patient's skin closely, as penetration depths can vary. I worry about the burns that could result from consumers applying these extremely powerful exfoliants by themselves. As I said in Chapter 1, more isn't always better—sometimes it's damaging.

A glycolic acid concentration around 8 percent is plenty for the face on a daily basis. You can use various strengths on the body, depending on the thickness and quality of the tissue. A 10 percent product might be fine on your chest, for example. Only doctors can use a single acid in an amount over 10 percent.

Regardless of their potency, all chemical exfoliants need to be buffered by a soothing ingredient that's also an anti-inflammatory. Some to look for on the label are aloe or cucumber. Almost every mainstream beauty range includes products with acid concentrations up to 10 percent in its line-up. More often than not, these items are formulated with a cream base, which has the added benefit of protecting the skin.

Ask the Doctor: *Should I stop exfoliating during the summer because my skin is protecting me from the sun?*

While it's true that surplus surface cells offer a slight shield against the rays, that benefit is outweighed by the greater gain you'll get in encouraging cell turnover. Yes, you need to be fastidious about applying sunblock to polished skin, but sunblock is much, much more effective at guarding you from UV-induced cell damage than the most concentrated layer of dead cells would ever be. There's really no way around it—you must slather on sun protection, especially from May through September.

COMMANDMENT 6: THOU SHALT EAT A HEALTHY, BALANCED DIET—AND DRINK LOTS OF WATER

When you go on any nutritional plan that restricts entire food groups, you're putting your health at risk. Sailors in the 1700s developed scurvy, after all, by not getting sufficient amounts of vitamin C. Meat-centric meals loaded with fatty acids rev up the skin and can lead to inflammation. In general, what's good for the heart is good for the skin. Following the guidelines for heart-healthy eating—green leafy vegetables, fresh fruit, lean meat—benefits your external appearance. You'll ensure that you get enough nutrients for general well-being, as well as for fit skin.

Water is also a key component to beautiful skin. You're not going to erase dry, flaky patches on your cheeks by downing gallons of water. You need a topical moisturizer to fix surface problems. But internal hydration aids cell and organ function and flushes waste products, important factors for healthy skin.

Ask the Doctor: *What effect does my diet have on my hair?*

Proper eating has a positive impact on your hair, there's no doubt. If you're stressed nutritionally, your body responds by shutting down certain mechanisms. When there's only a limited amount of nutrients available, your internal systems aren't going to waste that fuel producing new hair strands. Start taking care of yourself, and you'll be rewarded with thicker, stronger hair that grows faster.

COMMANDMENT 7: THOU SHALT SLATHER ON SUCH ANTIOXIDANTS AS VITAMINS C AND E OR GREEN TEA EVERY DAY

Free radicals, those molecules that assault and break down skin's supporting framework, are formed by oxidization. Think about the way a sliced apple turns brown if you leave it sitting on your kitchen counter or how rust forms on an old car bumper. Both are the result of oxidization. When an atom or ion loses an electron, it becomes a free radical: an unstable element that starts to pummel molecules surrounding it in an effort to regain the missing electron. Pollution, UV light, and stress are just a few of the entities that create free radicals. They're even discharged by the simple act of respiration.

POWER PLAYERS

My antioxidant hit list:

Alpha-lipoic acid
Beta-carotene
Carnitine (ergothioneine and thiotaine)
Coenzyme Q10 (idebenone)
Ferulic acid
Flavonoid
Grape seed extract (polyphenol and resveratrol)
Green tea
Isoflavone
Lutein
Lycopene
Milk thistle (silymarin)
Rosemary
Vitamin C
Vitamin E
White tea
Zinc

Obviously you can't eliminate your exposure to the little tyrants entirely. The good news is that you have antioxidants on your side to help you out. Antioxidants, like vitamins C and E and green tea (there's a broader list on the previous page), work by plugging the hole left by the liberated electron, effectively neutralizing the damage-inducing molecule. This frees the body of the stressors that slow its function and make it more sluggish. In addition to the diet plentiful in the antioxidant-rich foods I mentioned earlier, you'll need to take a topical approach to your antioxidants. As you now know, there's zero blood flow to the outermost layer of tissue. There's simply no way you could eat enough oranges in a day, for example, to get the equivalent skin effect of a coat of vitamin C serum. I'm such a believer in the beneficial effects of topical antioxidants that I rub them into my skin three times daily. Even applying them once a day (don't forget your body) will help keep your skin beaming and robust.

COMMANDMENT 8: THOU SHALT NOT BE AFRAID OF PIGMENT-REDUCING CREAMS; USE THEM DAILY

The technology in pigment-minimizing products is improving. What we had available to us a number of years ago was very limited—hydroquinone was the mainstay. We know now that hydroquinone, also an ingredient in photo developer, can be irritating. Pregnant women shouldn't use it because a certain amount can be absorbed internally. Today, there are a lot more options (some of them botanical), all sold over the counter, usually labeled as lighteners or brighteners. We've found that thyme has antipigment capabilities. Licorice extract and mulberry are two others shown to be effective. Despite the fact that some of these are foods, just as with antioxidants, you don't want to rely on diet alone to solve the problem. In large enough quantities, some could be toxic when ingested.

All these ingredients work at different points in the melanin production cycle. Some disperse existing patches of pigment. Others suppress melanin formation by blocking the melanocytes that synthesize it (Retin-A also has this effect). It's smart to select a topical with a variety of additives, so that you get the maximum benefit. Smooth these multifunctioning lotions on your face, hands, and body areas, such as the chest, where you may notice an abundance of dark patches. Follow with a layer of sunblock, as UV rays

---

BRIGHT SPOTS

Key ingredients for breaking up dark patches:
- Arbutin
- Azelaic acid
- Carnitine (ergothioneine and thiotaine)
- Kojic acid
- Licorice
- Mulberry
- Phyllanthus emblica
- Sepiwhite
- Thyme
- Waltheria

activate pigment cells, counteracting the effects of your pigment reducer.

Ask the Doctor: *Do I apply my lightening lotion solely on brown spots?*

Pigment-reducing creams do more than simply break up mottled areas. They also help regulate overall melanin production. For this reason, you should smooth your cream over your entire face, chest, and any other surface you feel is prone to spots. Since melanin is manufactured below the skin's surface, it could be developing but not yet visible. If you used your lotion only on what you could see, you'd miss the chance to stop the new stuff from forming.

THE HORMONE CONNECTION

Melasma, often called the mask of pregnancy, appears as diffuse, dark patches on the skin. Hormones trigger the condition, which means that it could even develop in birth control pill users. (Those on the pill may want to talk to their doctor about switching formulations, as that can often eliminate melasma.) Internal forces stimulate melasma-related pigment output, but the sun exacerbates the situation. Dissolving irregular areas with a cream or even a laser won't prevent them from reappearing, especially if you're regularly outdoors without SPF. In addition to sunblock, you'll need to slather on a product that suppresses melanin formation and keep it up until your hormone levels return to normal.

Pregnant women and new mothers always need to be careful and check a product's ingredients with their doctor.

Reality Show

Jean, 28, business analyst

I made an appointment with Dr. Copeland because my skin tone was uneven, and I had some brown patches, especially on my forehead and cheeks. I'm a woman of color, so you might not think that these dark spots would be noticeable on my skin, but they were. I was hesitant to use something as drastic as a laser on the discoloration, specifically because of my skin tone. She suggested I try her Pigment Formula lotion twice a day and her Microdermabrasion Formula scrub weekly.

The lotion, in particular, really seemed to have an effect. Within two weeks, I had started to see results. I've continued to use it, and my skin tone has evened out. I'm very happy with the way things have gone. I thought that since I had darker skin, I'd always have these little bits of excess pigment. Now I know that's not the case.

COMMANDMENT 9: THOU SHALT MAKE ANTIAGING CREAMS AND SERUMS YOUR NEW BEST FRIENDS AND APPLY THEM AT LEAST ONCE A DAY

After your preventative antioxidants and antipigment lotions are in place, it's time to address some of the skin damage that's already been done. As you get older, your skin needs more repair. Antiagers are sort of like a construction manager, who organizes and assigns builders to go in and reinforce a house's framework. But besides fixing things, these products minimize the chance of future breakdowns. I doubt that there's a man or woman out there who wouldn't like to have more of the collagen and elastin fibers that hold up tissue and keep it tight. Creating those strands requires an antiaging cream. The ingredients rev skin's growth process up a notch or two.

Soy, peptides, hyaluronic acid, selenium, and retinoids are just a few of my favorites. Oxidative damage increases with age. Since antioxidants help reduce this stress, they can also be considered antiaging. Many, including alpha-lipoic acid, coenzyme Q10, and thiotaine, have the added power to firm the tissue.

No single magic ingredient can do everything, so look for a topical with multiple youth builders. As I pointed out earlier, make sure they're near the top of the ingredient panel. Your serum won't be nearly as potent otherwise.

Ask the Doctor: *What are MMPs?*

Skin regenerates itself, and it degrades itself. As we age, collagen is particularly prone to the latter part of this cycle. Matrix metalloproteinase (MMP) is the enzyme involved in this collagen destruction. It would be great if we could find a way to prevent it from attaching to skin fibers. Scientists haven't been able to do that yet, but they're trying.

Ask the Doctor: *How old should I be to use an antiaging product?*

When your skin starts looking dull, it's time. An anti-aging cream is not preventative; antioxidants, sun-block, and healthy living are preventative. If you keep your collagen and elastin strong and protected, you may be able to go quite some time before you need to bring in the bigger guns.

JUST DO IT

One debate I often see playing out in magazines is whether it's more beneficial to exercise at the beginning of the day or at the end. What seems to makes the most sense is that people who find a gym near their home or office are more likely to stick to a workout program since it's easy to get to. The key is going consistently, whether it's before you head to your morning meetings or during your lunch break. The same principle applies to caring for your skin. It does you no good if you can't follow a regimen. You need to be faithful in order for one to deliver results. If that means you rub everything on as you're getting ready for the day, that's fine. If before bed is better for you because you have more time, that's effective as well. The most consequential action is establishing a daily ritual. That's how you get the health benefits of exercise and also ensure that you'll see positive changes in your skin in eight weeks or less.

WEIGHT TRAINING

Subcutaneous fat makes the skin smoother. African, Asian, and Hispanic skins have greater amounts of this type of tissue, so they often appear less wrinkled than Caucasians. But no matter what your genetic heritage, if you drop a lot of weight as a result of diet or exercise and turn yourself into skin and bones, your tissue isn't going to be soft and supple. You'll certainly have more crevices on your face. It's an extreme scenario but one that I see often enough that it's worth highlighting.

By the same token, constantly losing and then regaining weight will eventually stretch out your skin and exacerbate sagging. There are a lot of yo-yo dieters in my practice with this problem. Once you reach a size that's comfortable, as well as healthy, do whatever it takes to stay there. For one thing, you'll need only a single set of clothes. But more important, maintaining weight will have innumerable benefits to your skin's appearance and to the way it ages.

COMMANDMENT 10: THOU SHALT NOT SMOKE

Set aside all the problems that smoking can cause to your general health—emphysema, lung cancer, should I continue?—and think of its visible translation to your appearance. Smoking causes vasoconstriction of the tiny vessels that feed the skin, so the tissue isn't able to mend itself properly. Carbon monoxide and pollutants from cigarettes enter the pores and seep into the microcirculation, impeding skin's ability to oxygenate the dermis, which is where the new skin cells grow. The result is a complexion that's dull as opposed to luminous.

Smoking also surrounds the head in a huge free-radical cloud that strikes and degrades skin fibers, deepening lines and creating furrows. There are so many reasons to quit smoking. Whether you decide to do it for health reasons or for vanity, it doesn't matter—just break the bad habit.

PLANNING AHEAD

I've gone over the basics, and I've laid out the some general pitfalls that could have thrown you off track. Achieving true Creamy skin takes more than good habits and healthy living, however (although those are very important factors). The necessary push into the Creamy realm comes from repeating my five exercises or CEAMP. What are those? See the next page to discover the core of **The Beautiful Skin Workout**.

Chapter 3

The Five Exercises or CEAMP

There are so many things I love about my job: smoothing a noticeable bump in a woman's nose, thereby increasing her self-confidence, or giving a man some motivation to continue with his newly adopted healthy lifestyle by erasing his persistent love handles. But even though I am a plastic surgeon, I spend my days doing more than working with scalpels and cannulas in the operating room. I'm equally concerned with the quality of the skin itself, not just the ways I can shape it.

Here's the thing: I can't give a woman the firm, smooth, lifted face she wants if the tissue I have to work with is dull, crepey, dry, and discolored. As much as I pull and lift, if the texture and quality of skin are not addressed, the result of any procedure isn't going to make the person appear youthful and vibrant. Skin has internal and external components. They don't function independently, and a doctor can't treat them as separate entities if she wants to help the patient look his or her best. The entire system needs to be taken into account to ensure the best outcome.

CLOSE ENCOUNTERS

I've seen new patients who aren't plastic surgery first-timers. Sometimes they've had only one thing tweaked—their upper eyelids, for example. In other situations, they've undergone "the works"—eyes, cheeks, nose, and forehead—before booking an appointment with me. The one thing that these people have in common is that, despite the operations, they're still not happy. I'm sure they all appear younger than they did a year ago, but they don't look pretty. Their skin lacks freshness, and they seem old.

When I evaluate their faces, I tell them exactly why no surgery will correct the problems we both see: Their skin is in terrible shape. It could be vertical grooves above the upper lip, horizontal lines running across the forehead, or blotchy, mottled patches dotting their complexion. Those are all signs of a person with a lot of unhealthy habits, like heavy smoking, unrepentant sunbathing, or a diet consisting solely of cheese fries and chocolate layer cake.

Pulled skin does not magically become baby skin when the tissue in question is leathery. If a supple, radiant complexion is what you're after, I can tell you right now that you're not realistically going to attain that simply by entering the OR. Many people don't realize that while surgery can—quite effectively—remedy larger problems, like sagging jowls or puffy lower lids, it can't erase some other imperfections, such as fine lines around the mouth or rough texture. The good news is that those are problems *you* can fix. You don't have to settle for a dull, lackluster complexion now that effective skin care has gone mainstream and potent products are widely available. With the help of **The Beautiful Skin Workout**, you can, and should, strive to be Creamy.

Ask the Doctor: *If I don't jump straight into the entire program, will I still need only eight weeks to arrive at Creamy skin?*

It's okay to start slowly if you're timid, but it's going to take you longer than eight weeks to reach your goal. Say you're a couch potato who doesn't even walk to the store. If the extent of your exercise is to get in your car, stroll around the supermarket, then drive home, you won't run a mile on your first attempt. But by pushing yourself every day, instead of just a couple of times a week, you'll complete that distance in short order. Think of your progression to Creamy skin in the same terms.

Reality Show

Alice, 43, bartender

I grew up in California and spent a lot of time in the sun. During my twenties and thirties, my skin was fine, but when I turned forty, everything changed. Suddenly, my face had areas of mottled discoloration, concentrated under my eyes and on

A SIMPLE PLAN

The heart of **The Beautiful Skin Workout** is the five exercises below. Ideally, you'd go through the program twice a day, every day. (If you can do it only once daily, that's fine; it will just require more time to see a change in your skin.) Each step has a specific effect, from increasing your skin's health to eliminating wrinkles. This regimen is so easy to follow, it can be summed up in five letters: CEAMP.

 Cleanse

 Exfoliate

 Activate

 Moisturize

 Protect

my cheeks. If I got a pimple or a scratch, the area would turn really dark and scar. Everything showed up. It was a nightmare.

I work long nights behind a bar, which does my skin no favors. I'd gone to dermatologists for microdermabrasion treatments, which made me look more refreshed but did nothing about my complexion's color, tone, pigmentation, or scarring.

Until that point, I'd never done much more than wash my face. Since my skin is oily, I didn't apply moisturizer or anything else. I thought that I didn't need it. Then, all of a sudden, I really, really did need it. After several people I didn't know came up to me and offered numbers for dermatologists, I decided to take action. I went to Dr. Copeland, and she immediately put me on a new skin-care regimen.

I became addicted to going through the whole CEAMP routine. Even if I get home dead tired at four-thirty in the morning, I always cleanse, exfoliate, treat, and moisturize. I'm religious about applying my pigment-lightening lotion and smoothing on eye cream. Keeping with the program makes a big difference. I saw results instantly. Within a few months, you could do a serious before-and-after photo session with me. The change in my skin is just amazing.

I feel so much better about myself now, too. Before, I was obsessed with glancing in the mirror to see how bad my skin was. I spackled on lots of heavy concealer and worried about what other people thought of me. Not anymore. I can breeze into my job and trust that I look great.

STEP 1: CLEANSE

 The surface of your face and body is home to millions of bacteria. Before you get completely grossed out and run screaming toward a vat of disinfectant, keep in mind that certain types of bacteria are good and beneficial. But invariably, some of the ones that aren't make their way

READING MATERIALS

Product manufacturers are required to list ingredients in order of their relative quantity; how much of one additive is in a formula compared with the others. Suppose you are looking for something made with the antioxidant vitamins C and E. If you find them at the bottom of the inventory, there's the least amount of those two vitamins in relation to everything else in that cleanser or lotion. Conversely, if paraben, a preservative, is the first thing on the label, it has the highest concentration.

When I buy anything, from a new tube of mascara to a loaf of bread, I always read the ingredient panel, and I think that's a good thing. You don't need to be a biochemist to pick out certain ingredients to avoid: fragrances, dyes, and forms of silicone. They don't increase an item's efficacy, so it doesn't make sense to put an unnecessary element on your skin. In addition, check to be sure that your skin-care items have been allergy tested.

through tiny cracks in the tissue. They work themselves inside your body, where they can start an infection. I already told you that this is the reason you should avoid harsh scrubbing items, such as loofah brushes, which can scratch the skin. There's no need to increase the number of tissue fissures and give unhealthy bacteria more entranceways. But occasionally, small openings can develop naturally, usually the result of simple, environmentally induced wear and tear. For that reason, it helps to be vigilant about ridding yourself of the bad bacteria sitting on top of your face and body.

Ask the Doctor: *If my facial wash is allergy tested, I don't have to worry about anything bad happening, right?*

Allergy testing doesn't guarantee that no one will get a reaction. It indicates that the product was tried on a number of random people and no member of that group had an adverse response. If thirty testers are unaffected, that's pretty good. Unfortunately, extremely sensitive skin might still get irritated, even if the cream in question has been certified as allergy tested. Those types should be careful.

THIS IS HOW WE DO IT

The act of massage is therapeutic. Each and every one of my patients receives a lymphatic massage after surgery because the treatment helps healing. Stimulating the lymph system increases circulation and reduces waste products, swelling, and inflammation. It also brings in the powerhouses that the cells use to care for themselves. If you massage your skin with your fingertips while you cleanse your face, not only will you feel more relaxed, you'll also be benefiting your complexion.

Since an important aspect of taking care of your face and body is to keep the tissue firm and uplifted, don't tug in a downward direction when you wash. Gravity goes toward the floor; you should aim for the ceiling. Work your facial cleanser in a soothing upward motion from your chin to your forehead. Use firm, upward strokes when washing your body as well.

WATER TESTING

While plain H_2O is good for you internally and externally, minerals in water can be damaging to skin. The difference between hard and soft water relates to the mineral content of what's coming out of the tap. There are fewer minerals in the soft variety, so there's less to irritate the face and body. These materials may also build up on hair. You'll frequently notice that your hair is shinier and has more bounce if you shampoo it in soft water.

The market is full of showerhead filters that supposedly strain out heavy minerals. If you live in an area supplied with hard water, you may want to consider installing a soft water purification system in your house as one effective way to block these particles. It will ensure that, whether you wash your hands in the kitchen or lather your face at the bathroom sink, you're not inflicting unnecessary minerals on the tissue.

Ask the Doctor: *I've heard that water dries skin. Is splashing my face a bad thing?*

Running water on its own is a lot less dehydrating than any chemical ever would be. Will H_2O break up grease on the skin's surface? No. To do that requires a compound able to dissolve the bonds fastening dirt and oil to the tissue. You need to wash with a cleanser, but a simple, quick blast of water won't negatively affect you.

EYE SCHOOL

Skin is not the same all over. There are more glands in the armpits, for example; the fingertips have thermoregulating mechanisms that aren't found in other body areas. Around the eyes, you should practice caution when applying items, such as fragrance, that could get in the lashes or the eye itself and trigger irritation. Creams and solutions may be marked if they're ophthalmologist tested, indicating that they are certified to be safe for use near the eye. Certain cleansers are formulated for the entire face, but in general, the eyes take a different kind of care.

The tissue is very delicate and thin. Rubbing and scrubbing to get rid of makeup will pull that fragile skin. Many brands of facial wash also dissolve eyeshadow, liner, and mascara. However, some types of mascara, particularly waterproof versions, are oil-based to keep their formulas from running (since eyes are wet). If your face product isn't easily lifting all traces of mascara, you may want to invest in a separate eye makeup remover. Like dissolves like, so oftentimes an oily cleanser will take off waterproof mascara without much effort on your part. Press a cotton pad saturated with remover to your closed eyelid. Allow the liquid to sit on the lashes, then swipe it off with a fresh, saturated cotton square.

 Ask the Doctor: *Do I really need a toner?*

Toners aren't just another unnecessary item that beauty companies are trying to sell you. The skin's surface should always be slightly acidic to keep harmful bacteria at bay. Toning liquids, in tandem with cleansers, help adjust skin's pH level to create the optimal environment for cellular growth and function. It's akin to breeding cells in a test tube. If the circumstances aren't right, they won't multiply. However, your toner should be gentle, with such ingredients as allantoin or sorbic acid, not harsh, skin-stripping additives like alcohol or witch hazel.

HEAVY-HANDED

I don't suggest thick creams as cleaners or moisturizers because they can potentially block pores. I had a patient who coated her face with Crisco. If you were stepping into the harsh cold and applied Crisco first, you'd actually be doing a good thing, since the shortening would act as a barrier. But slathering Crisco on every day as a matter of course is clogging. The skin is supposed to interact with your normal environment. It's designed to exchange oxygen, to perspire, and to rid itself of bacteria.

Think about the way you outfit yourself to venture into a thunderstorm. You put on your rubber raincoat and boots because they're impermeable to water and keep your body and feet dry as you're splashing through puddles on the way to your car. But if you wear your weather gear for a long time, you start to sweat underneath the protective layer. That's because your plastic wardrobe not only isn't letting any water in, it also keeps any air from getting out. Your body heat builds up inside your clothes and you perspire.

A heavy skin-care product is like a rubber raincoat. Yes, you're preventing some outside forces from reaching the skin (I say *some* because UV light can pass through the most occlusive ointment), but you're also not allowing the tissue to release what it needs to in order to maintain a nice, stable equilibrium.

Ask the Doctor: *I have oily skin. Will a toner containing alcohol help dry it out?*

If you have a greasy complexion, your goal is to reduce the flow of sebum making its way to the skin's surface. However, you won't accomplish that by dehydrating your face with alcohol. This only rids your skin of the oils sitting on top; it won't stop your glands from producing more. Continue to use an alcohol-free toner to maintain your skin's pH. You'll be able to regulate sebum flow with exfoliation, described in Step 2.

Ask the Doctor: *My pores are huge. How can I make them smaller?*

Just cleansing and toning your face will go a long way toward minimizing the appearance of your pores. They grow larger as we get older; it's part of the natural aging process. Despite what you may see in magazines or on television, pores are not valves. You can't simply open and close them at will. The holes do stretch, however, so if there's debris in one, it will be bigger. Empty the space of the large obstruction (by washing your face, *not* by picking at a blockage), and the skin returns to its previous size. Excess sebum can also magnify pores. Regulating oil flow, which consistent cleansing and toning—in addition to exfoliation—will do, helps the pores seem less noticeable. A clay-based mask acts like a poultice to draw dirt and oil out of large pores, particularly around the nose area. I suggest applying one weekly, if this is a concern of yours. After I perform a rhinoplasty and the splint is off, I have my patients return to their cleansing, toning, and mask routine. It really seems to speed healing and get those tissues to shrink to their normal size.

STEP 2: EXFOLIATE

Exfoliation is the surefire method for producing skin radiance, that lit-from-within-by-a-1,000-watt-bulb effect. Plastic surgeons have long known that by removing the top layer of skin, we can speed cellular turnover underneath. Sloughing off withered dead cells triggers the body mechanism that hatches new ones. There are many ways to exfoliate and even more opportunities to do it incorrectly.

As I've pointed out, the skin on your face and body isn't uniform; it thickens at differing rates. Think about calluses. Your feet may develop them, but your face doesn't. We're able to apply stronger, more aggressive exfoliating agents on the areas below the neck than we can above it. Regardless, no piece of your skin should flake or peel after you exfoliate. In the past, chemical peels sometimes caused

SCHEDULING CONFLICTS

There's a time and place for everything, including how often you should apply your exfoliators.

Chemical: Mild cream or serum formulations (acid concentrations of 10 percent or less) are safe to use twice a day, assuming your skin can tolerate it. However, your tissue needs at least a week between chemical peels whose acids are stronger than 10 percent to repair itself.

Physical: A gritty scrub should be pressed into service only once or twice weekly, three at most.

skin to shed visibly. But the lighter formulations we use today allow us to deliver the exfoliating benefits of older versions, without obvious flaking. Oftentimes, skin isn't even red after an in-office treatment, so a person can head straight back to work—hence, the procedure's nickname: "lunchtime peel."

Ask the Doctor: *Does my greasy complexion require a special exfoliant?*

I often suggest that patients with overly oily skin use salicylic acid to stimulate cell turnover. It's a good option because it's gentle and anti-inflammatory but still unplugs pores and manages cell function. I also recommend searching for a product containing sebum regulators. These ingredients even skin function, quieting oil production if the body is secreting excessive amounts or speeding things up if it's not producing enough.

PARTICLE THEORY

Microdermabrasion polishes are beneficial because they give you a physical exfoliation that's not too harsh and is bacteria-free. But at-home microdermabrasion machines are like loofah brushes: dirty. Unless you're aiming to torture your skin, avoid exfoliating with anything that doesn't rinse down the drain.

Of course, you still have to be careful when you use your hands to scrub your face. Don't press so hard that your complexion becomes raw and red. Remember to work the cream down your neck and chest and over your hands, especially if you have a lot of sun damage. Alligator or leathery skin could begin my program with microdermabrasion-type exfoliation, but suede skin probably doesn't need it. All things being equal, however, it's better to start out with a mild exfoliant and work up to something with more intensity.

Ask the Doctor: *Are microdermabrasion sessions and chemical peels safe outside of a physician's office?*

Like so many beauty treatments, microdermabrasion and peels used to be solely medical procedures and now they're widely available. When evaluating where to go, cleanliness should be one of your main criteria. It's a bacterial issue. When I perform microdermabrasion, I sterilize the machine's tip since it's pressing right up against the skin. Regardless of whether you choose a spa or a doctor's office, make sure the equipment is sanitary. You can't just go in and let people rub all over your face without knowing if the place is spotless.

The other thing to keep in mind is the level of training of the person who's administering the treatment. Two-day educational courses are available for most anything these days. A pediatrician could take a weekend class in breast augmentation, for example, then set up shop doing implants. It makes much more sense, if one is having plastic surgery, to go to a doctor who has spent years, not hours, studying in the field. By the same token, an aesthetician in a spa, even one run by an M.D., can't provide the same level of expertise as the physician himself or herself. My nurse has been in the operating room with me every day for six years. Can she perform the actual surgery? No. Unless you're doing something mild, you often need a practiced eye that knows how to deal with complications.

STOP SIGNS

Indications of overexfoliation:

Blotchiness
Irritation
Redness

DARK MARK

Aggressively polishing skin can cause changes in its coloring. This condition is known as postinflammatory hyperpigmentation. Excite the tissue, and the body brings in cells to calm it down. Sometimes, this mechanism goes overboard, and you develop brown spots. Certain people are more susceptible to that outcome than others. If you fall into that category, you already know because when you have a cut, it heals lighter or darker than the surrounding area. Be a little more aware before you start any exfoliation. You could test a product on your arm initially, then move to your face.

Ask the Doctor: *I had radiation treatments for cancer. Can I still follow your program?*

Radiated skin can be leathery, but as is the case with any specific need, you should to listen to your skin before treating it. I'd be especially careful to avoid fragrances

---

SLEIGHT OF HAND

A number of patients have told me that putting their glycolic acid–based exfoliating cream all over their hands has hardened their nail plates and made their cuticles look better. Their newly thickened nails also break and crack less as a result. It may be that the stimulation-by-exfoliation principle, which works so well on skin, has an additional beneficial effect on nail quality.

---

and other ingredients that could inflame the sensitive tissue. If you try one of these steps and have a problem, by all means, stop.

After radiation, your skin is probably dehydrated. Moisturization is the most important action for you. Begin simply by washing with nondrying cleanser and applying lotion. You could use an alpha hydroxy acid, but don't select a potent formulation. Microdermabrasion on a radiated chest isn't something to start with; it could be irritating. Right now, your skin is more susceptible to infection and doesn't have the reserves to combat aggravation, so you need to aid it as much as you can.

JUST FOR MEN

Shaving is a type of physical exfoliation, but one that can cause tiny skin breaks. You can't follow it straight away with a chemical exfoliant because your skin will be too sensitive and develop irritation and redness. If you shave in the morning, don't immediately slap on your acids or antioxidants—you'll feel the burn. You're obviously not going over your forehead, nose, and upper cheeks with a razor, though. Treat those sections first, then move to your cheeks before progressing with the rest of your CEAMP program.

 Ask the Doctor: *As I've gotten older, I've noticed that, while my skin has become thinner, I'm also developing thicker patches, similar to calluses, on my face and body. Will exfoliation remove them?*

Those areas of dense skin tissue are called keratoses. Cell turnover slows with time, so the cells themselves heap up on the surface, resulting in the condition you describe. The bad news is that keratoses become more plentiful as the years pass, as do brown spots. However, daily exfoliation will cut down on both their numbers.

Keratoses are often mistaken for precancerous lesions. If you exfoliate consistently, you'll make your skin more even and weed out the keratoses. Anything that remains could, in fact, be a precancerous lesion and should be evaluated by a qualified physician.

HAND-PICKED

If I could do one thing that would cure my acne patients of their skin woes, it would be to convince them to keep their hands away from their faces. The biggest problem people have with their skin is picking it. This traumatizes the tissue: Don't do it. I know sometimes people have a pimple or a clogged pore that they want to get rid of. They're desperate to squeeze their skin, so they pinch the area, causing a contusion and extending the zone of injury. When a doctor drains an abscess, she doesn't smash all the tissue surrounding it. The point is limiting the damage to the skin, not exacerbating it. The irony is that if you just leave your pimple alone, it will probably heal faster than it will once you perform self-surgery because you're causing the body less angst. Look at your skin first.

> ## BURN RATE
>
> Once you cause a hole by picking at your face, you create a little sore. You cannot put acid on it. Let me repeat that: You cannot put acid on an open wound. It's irritating, and it will burn. If you're plagued by breakouts, don't be rough on them. If you're reading this after you've already gone to town on your complexion, put a little occlusive antibacterial cream, such as Neosporin or Bacitracin, on those spots.

If it's not compromised, you could use an acid on the blemish to help speed its disappearance. It's also permissible to scrub with a physical exfoliant.

SPECIAL CASE SCENARIO

Retin-A is a form of vitamin A, which increases blood supply to the tissue and encourages cells to turn over. However, it's not an exfoliant like acids. That's a common misconception. Exfoliants sweep away dead cells. Retin-A doesn't do this. In fact, it actually has some antioxidant properties in that it neutralizes free radicals, in addition to its main function of encouraging cell growth.

The life cycle of a skin cell is the same in everyone, although it slows with age. Cells march up the ladder from the dermis, reach the surface, and then, boom, fall off the ladder. This progression signals the body to make more cells. When they collect on top instead, the message is: Stop manufacturing cells, we've got enough already.

If you remove this top layer, you're indirectly telling the dermis to produce cells. That's exfoliation. Retin-A also commands the body to form cells, but it does this by upping blood flow to the dermis, so that cells in the deepest skin layers are healthier and more active. Highly effective nonprescription forms of vitamin A, such as retinol, are now available. They give the body's cell factory instructions similar to the doctor-dispensed version of vitamin A.

Ask the Doctor: *If Retin-A is good for my face, should I use it on the rest of my body?*

The body needs vitamin A. Studies have shown that Retin-A improves wound healing and the quality of collagen. It's fine to use Retin-A everywhere, but it's ex-

---

BIRDS OF A FEATHER

Men and women frequently ask me if there's a difference between Renova and Retin-A. The creamy vehicle that contains the vitamin A in Renova is less irritating than the oil-free gel with which the original Retin-A Micro is made. However, the Renova manufacturers added a perfume when they created their offshoot. I very rarely prescribe it because I don't like fragranced skin care.

---

pensive. A prescription topical has a higher concentration of vitamin A than an over-the-counter cream does. But we've learned that it's not necessary to have vitamin A at a prescription level to get its positive effect.

Ten years ago, every single one of my patients, including myself, was on Retin-A. It was all we had. Today, I don't use Retin-A; I get vitamin A through other topicals. My skin is still Creamy. People with acne and overactive sebaceous glands may require the little bit of extra strength available in a prescription. However, antiaging benefits can be had without that amount of intensity.

AT FIRST BLUSH

People with rosacea have sensitive skin, in addition to a problem with inflammation. Those with psoriasis, eczema, or flaky, scaly tissue have to tread lightly as well. Exfoliating could convince the cells to function in a more rhythmic, therapeutic way. But sometimes that stimulation turns the skin blotchy and red. When I see someone with rosacea, I have him go more slowly through **The Beautiful Skin Workout**, but he can absolutely follow the basic outline. If he can stick to it, his skin is going to be clearer and better than it's ever been.

Ask the Doctor: *May I combine my cleansing step with the exfoliating one by using a face wash containing scrubbing beads?*

Since cleansing can rob the skin of the oils and nutrients that it needs, you always want that process to be gentle. Washing with an abrasive product twice a day is definitely too harsh. By the same token, you shouldn't be using a physical exfoliant daily, either.

STEP 3: ACTIVATE

 We're now at the midway point of **The Beautiful Skin Workout**, and it's your opportunity to take prime advantage of the technological advances in skin-care research and development. There's absolutely no good reason for you not to slather yourself with antioxidants and antiaging topicals. If you've mistreated your face and body in the past, now is your chance to undo the damage. It's almost hard to avoid antioxidants, as the free-radical zappers are in literally everything these days, from face cream and foundation to sunblock and self-tanner. Forms of my A-listers can be found at varying price points, from the drugstore aisle to the department store counter.

The preceding exfoliant step plays an important part in how the powerful components of this third stage perform. A product will be unevenly distributed if you apply it to flaky tissue, because the surface isn't smooth. By putting on antioxidants and antiagers after you've polished your skin, you allow their active ingredients to penetrate deeper into the tissue for a long-lasting, glowing effect. If you're trying to wipe out excessively discolored patches, apply an antipigment lotion during Step 3 as well.

OH, SAY CAN YOU C?

It's a catch-22: The forms of vitamin C that are easily absorbed by the body also break down quickly in product formulations. Developers have discovered, however, that combining the powerful antioxidant with another ingredient, like glycolic acid, may increase the amount of vitamin C that permeates the tissue. You don't need to be mixing up fresh vitamin C from powder in your own little home lab to have Creamy skin, though. For one thing, the powder that you're blending might not have a chemical configuration that's amenable to skin. Freshness isn't really the issue, in terms of whether or not your vitamin C sinks into skin. As long as vitamin C is an ingredient in your serum, and you use the product in a timely manner—as opposed to letting it sit on the bathroom shelf for months—the item you're smoothing on should be beneficial to your face and body.

EYE WAYS

When you're applying creams and serums around the eye, be cautious. Even products that are allergy tested might not agree with everyone, and the eye area swells faster than other locations on the body. Start by tapping your skin-care product on a little bit low, closer to the cheekbone. Once you're sure that it's not going to trigger an adverse reaction, you may choose to use it across your upper eyelids, as well as on the skin around the eye socket, so that all of the tissue is healthy and supple.

A COMPLEX ISSUE

New miracle age-reversing ingredients are hitting the market all the time. The most overwhelming part of the whole thing is that the claims behind these magic mixtures aren't backed by the same real science that's used, for example, to test a new drug for the heart. Beauty companies often create their own proprietary, patented hybrids, which no one else can duplicate. Those can be confusing because no one else really knows what's in the product. Secret blends aren't necessarily any better than the ones made with the components we already know are effective: antioxidants and antiaging preparations.

Ask the Doctor: *Should my antiaging cream contain growth hormone?*

As a physician, I'm not comfortable with adding growth hormone to topical skin care. No double-blind, placebo-controlled, long-term studies have shown that growth hormone is safe, so scientists have been unable to draw any definitive conclusions. If it actually does stimulate cell multiplication when applied to skin, who's to say that only healthy cells would proliferate? There's always a concern, when you're talking about encouraging cellular production, that you could trigger a cellular overgrowth, such as cancer. We're also not certain how additional growth hormone could affect the levels of other hormones. Eventually, it's possible that researchers will develop a safe, thoroughly evalu-

A SURGEON'S SECRETS FOR SCAR PREVENTION

Yes, my patients typically come to see me because they want to improve their looks. You could have guessed that. But they have another desired outcome from their surgery that, while secondary, is almost as important as ending up with a newly defined jawline: People rarely want anyone else to know that they've gone under the knife.

Massage is one of my tricks for ensuring that my patients don't end up with telltale post-op marks. You can employ some of the same principles if you nick your shin or cut your forearm. As always, there's a balance between stimulating and irritating the body. Massage helps remodel and soften the collagen in scars. However, you don't want to manipulate the area around a wound, so you have to wait for it to seal before you start your rubdowns.

Silicone seems to quell scar formation. While I'm not generally a silicone proponent, this is one situation in which silicone patches or ointments may be therapeutic. Never, ever put acids or even regular, plain moisturizers on open skin. They can cause harm because they're formulated to be applied to the surface of the epidermis, not the dermal tissue underneath. In addition, since exposed patches are missing their barrier layer, they're prone to infection.

Your injured area shouldn't be dry or wet: Keep it protected. Cover it with a Band-Aid, but at the same time, make sure the section is lubricated enough to be conducive to healing. An antibiotic ointment, like Neosporin or Bacitracin, functions as both a protective layer and a repair agent. Don't let a cut dehydrate to the point that its edges begin to pucker; this prevents the developing collagen from laying flat. Scar formation can increase pigment production, so it's often helpful to apply a pigment-reducing lotion. Again, wait until the wound has closed.

ated form of this hormone for use in skin care. Until they do, there are plenty of good ingredients, which are already proven safe; we don't need to play around with potentially harmful additives with no benefits.

RELAXED FEELING

The Botox a doctor injects in forehead furrows and crow's feet doesn't make the recipient's skin young and healthy; it just helps it appear less wrinkled. That's no substitute for Creamy skin. If you'd like to minimize fine lines but you're not ready to dabble in cosmetic procedures, topical Botox-like creams are great additions to the Activate step. Just keep your expectations in check. There are chemical compounds, such as argeriline, pentapeptides, GABA, and DMAE, which can relax the little nerve endings in skin to give the entire complexion an immediate smoothness. There's nothing wrong with that. These products can go where the needle can't, like close to the lashes and delicate lid tissue. If you can't afford injections or if you bruise easily and, therefore, avoid needles, a topical relaxer can be a wonderfully effective alternative.

The nice thing about this family of ingredients is that they give the skin and the psyche an instant boost. You will notice marked improvement five minutes after you rub in a cream. It's like a miracle. When you go on a diet and step on the scale after one day, if you've already lost a pound, you're that much more motivated to stick with your new eating plan. Who can't benefit from a little positive reinforcement? Even though these topicals won't

FACE FACTS

Monthly facials may have a positive impact on your skin, if the treatments relax you and contribute to your overall sense of well-being. But you're not going to end up with Creamy skin by taking care of your face only one day out of thirty. If you're on a limited budget, I suggest putting your money into something that you'll do every day: your skin-care routine.

stimulate collagen production or make your skin healthy, seeing wrinkles swiftly disappear is very satisfying in itself.

BODY OF EVIDENCE

Be sure to use antioxidants and antiagers under your chin. Skin on the face and hands is frequently exposed, whereas the rest of a person is usually covered. Those protected areas won't age at the same rate as the ones subjected daily to the sun, wind, and pollution. Definitely coat vitamin serums down your neck and chest and on your hands. Unless money is no object, you're probably not going to treat your legs and stomach with the same items, because those types of products are fairly expensive. In this situation, I give you permission to combine Step 3 with Step 4: Moisturize. A cost-effective solution is to find a fragrance-free body lotion containing vitamin C and other antiagers.

TOUCH AND GO

For the myriad ways that antioxidant and antiaging serums improve skin tissue, you actually need very little of them to have a positive impact. You certainly don't have to glob these products all over your face and body. For one thing, it may take them a while to dry, and no one wants to waste a lot of time standing around waiting for that to happen. Just make sure that you get your antioxidants and antiagers on your skin; that's the most important part.

Reality Show

Samantha, 34, nurse

Growing up, I never had a problem with my skin. No one in my family had acne, so I guess I just assumed that I'd always have a clear complexion. But when I moved to New York City from Florida, I started breaking out all along my jawline. It was bad. I have to pull my hair back for my job, which exposed my acne even more. The situation was awful, and I was so paranoid.

I take care of myself by exercising and making proper food choices. When you see someone with bad skin, you often think that she's eating junk food, but that wasn't the case with me, which was sad. When I went to see Dr. Copeland, she told me that I wasn't cleansing well, so the bacteria were getting back in. My face was really sensitive at first, so I could use only her Daily Cleanser and Normalizing Toner and Advanced Acne Formula. Within six to eight weeks, my skin was so, so much better.

Now I'm applying everything, including her Pigment Formula. My acne scars and dark spots have disappeared, and I get compliments on my skin all the time. I'm back in Florida now. You can't wear makeup here because it melts right off. I'm just thrilled when I look at my bare face.

STEP 4: MOISTURIZE

 For skin that feels like satin, hydration is the key. As I've said, what you do for your body internally is as important as your actions on its surface. The visible layer of skin doesn't receive any blood, meaning it gets no nutrients. You're the one responsible for making the tissue soft and plump by regularly applying lotion. In fact, this simple act often causes fine lines to disappear temporarily because the extra moisture swells the tissue. I've seen patients shun hydrators because they're afraid they'll make their skin greasy or lead to a breakout. With the correct formulation, this is simply not the case.

IT TAKES TWO

Moisturizers fall into two main categories: humectant and lubricant. Hyaluronic acid is one commonly used humectant and is also naturally present in skin tissue.

WATCH LIST

Certain common face and body moisturizers can negatively impact some skins types:

Lanolin: This ingredient can be irritating and also a little heavy.

Mineral and coconut oils: These often clog pores.

Nut oils: If you have allergies, these formulas may cause an adverse reaction.

Silicone and its other forms, such as dimethicone: These chemical compounds are notorious pore blockers.

Humectants work by drawing water from the air and on the skin's surface into the epidermal cells, keeping them bouncy and moist. That's their job. So in between rubbing in your face cream and your sunblock, you might mist your skin with a little mineral-free water. It will give the humectants on your skin that much more H_2O to absorb and plump the tissue, minimizing the appearance of wrinkles.

Lubricants act as an extra protective layer on skin. They trap existing water in the cells. While they don't let the hydrogen and oxygen molecules escape, they also don't bring anything in to help the current situation. If you were going out into a harsh climate, you'd be wise to wear this additional shield. Olive oil, which is made up of beneficial polyphenols and fatty acids, is one good lubricating ingredient for the body.

FRINGE BENEFITS

Alpha hydroxy acids help the skin work better, which may improve your body's natural hydration process. As you follow all the steps in **The Beautiful Skin Workout**, you might find that you're able to taper off the amount of moisturizer you use.

MISTAKEN IDENTITY

People can have oily complexions that are still flaky and rough. An exfoliant, such as alpha hydroxy acid, can help normalize skin texture, but moisturizer is also necessary—even for those who get pimples. What the majority of men and women don't understand is that hydrating means bringing water, not oil, back into skin. Its purpose is to keep the keratin cells from getting desiccated and dried out (which contributes to flaking). You don't need oil to hydrate. The oil in a lotion simply acts as a protective mechanism. Humectants are what ward off dehydration, and there are products containing them that won't trigger breakouts.

PLACE IN TIME

Your skin has different needs depending on the month. During the summer, the glands produce more oil, so I'd switch to a product that's not as moisturizing. The zone around the nose and down toward the mouth contains a lot of glands, so you probably want to go easy on it all year-round. But you don't have the same kind of glands in the hands or legs, for example, so those areas frequently flake and scale, regardless of the season.

 Ask the Doctor: *If I have greasy skin, should I be using a moisturizer?*

Yes, although you probably don't need that much. An oil-free product is probably a better choice if you have overactive skin. Be careful where you apply it. You don't need to slap it all over your face; just target the areas that are usually dry.

FAUX NATURAL

It amazes me that so many products are called natural and yet are formulated with silicone and dimethicone. Those are compound polymers derived from oils and greases. Their purpose is to give skin an immediate smoothness by coating it with a layer of slick particles. It also reduces some visible signs of aging because it fills grooves around the mouth, eyes, and forehead. However, that silky, plump surface is fleeting. It disappears as soon as you wash your face. This book is not about cosmetics, nor is it about faking your way to a better complexion. There's no reason to make skin look good if it's not healthy. And why have your face appear youthful for a few hours, if as soon as you get undressed, you reveal a wrinkly old body? If you remain faithful to **The Beautiful Skin Workout**, you will be rewarded with genuinely Creamy skin from top to bottom.

HEY, BIG SPENDER

You've probably heard the youth-restoring promises of skin-care companies pushing pricey, naturally sourced, antiaging ingredients, such as caviar, and wondered if the claims were true. Yes, fish eggs are filled to bursting with fatty acids and vitamins. But do they do anything more than a product made with fatty acids and vitamins derived from a less-expensive place? The answer is no. Plus, to mask caviar's fishy smell, the manufacturers have to add a lot of fragrance to the final formula. And we know that perfumes aren't beneficial in skin care. Some caviar is better than others. How do you know that you're even getting the good stuff?

Bovine placenta is another nontraditional extract, which is very rich in nutrients and also extremely expensive. Does it work any better at revitalizing skin than a regular product? Probably not. When you're evaluating antiaging creams, stick to ones with ingredients that are basic and make sense. I promise, you won't get taken to the cleaners.

LIP SERVICE

Tissue around the month is unique. For one thing, it's very thin (lips appear red because you're seeing the blood flow underneath). It's also generally more sensitive, as well as more absorbent, than other body surfaces. As a result, you need special products to treat it.

The CEAMP program is still effective on this area. Moisturization and protection are especially critical. We often wet our lips, which makes them more prone to cracking. UV rays and stress can trigger the formation of cold sores, which are related to the herpes simplex virus to which many people are exposed. The virus often lies dormant, but it can flare up when provoked by sunlight, emotional stress, and illness. By caring for the skin around the lips, you'll minimize the chances of this happening.

Antioxidants and exfoliants, such as glycolic acid, are great ideas, as are occlusive lubricants and SPF. Just be sure to check the label in advance: Since we often end up ingesting lip balms, anything you use needs to be proven safe when taken internally.

Ask the Doctor: *I have terrible lines around my mouth. Can a topical get rid of them?*

Wrinkles surrounding the lips are some of the most difficult to treat. Following the CEAMP program will definitely help improve the quality of the tissue, which can reduce the look of these fine lines. Topical Botox-like creams are also beneficial, as they may help soften grooves. However, it's important to be realistic. Complete eradication of issues concerning the lip skin will probably require a trip to the doctor's office for some laser resurfacing and/or filler injections.

Ask the Doctor: *What can I do topically to increase the size of my thin lips?*

There are three methods for plumping skinny lips without injections of a filler. One: Exfoliate and hydrate to get rid of flaking and allow the lips to retain moisture. Mild glycolic or lactic acids do an effective job on this area. Two: Try a product that increases blood flow temporarily to the mouth. Ingredients like cinnamon and nicotinic acid work as vasodilators to open the blood vessels and swell the lips right away. Three: Look for items containing lipoic acid, vitamin C, or other ingredients that help build collagen over time. These won't deliver an immediate effect, but with continued use, they will help give lips a longer-lasting size increase.

We should expect topical lip plumpers to do more than simply inflate the tissue. They should have the same quality and effectiveness as antiaging face creams and make the skin healthier, smoother, and softer.

WARNING

Never put anything on your lips containing camphor. Camphor is a form of benzene. Benzenes are chemicals that are toxic and carcinogenic. Manufacturers often use camphor in balms and ointments the same way they do menthol, but it's not good to breathe it in or ingest it, despite its cooling sensation. How camphor is allowed in a preparation, even in minute amounts, I do not know. I would definitely steer clear of it.

Reality Show

Susan, 40, musician

The only thing I used to put on my face was soap that I purchased at the drugstore. I've never been a frou-frou person. My dad had bad skin, so I figured it was genetic. Of course, my face looked really good if I put makeup on it, but underneath it was ruddy and prone to breakouts. Dr. Copeland told me that I ought to have a peaches-and-cream complexion, not a red one, and it was actually possible for me to achieve that.

It felt weird to pay attention to what I was applying to my face and to take the time to use all the products. But I was tired of having good skin one day and bad the next; I wanted consistency. After a few weeks, my face was looking just as Dr. Copeland promised—smooth and blemish free. Her Rewind Reparative Night Serum is fantastic. I put it around my mouth and the texture is so much better.

You get in the habit of self-confidence when your face is always clear. You're no longer trying to hide anything on your complexion. That's a nice feeling.

STEP 5: PROTECT

 The fountain of youth is neither exclusive nor difficult to find; it's sitting on the shelves of your neighborhood beauty aisles: SPF. Sun exposure, unlike your genetic code, is controllable and one of the major factors in determining

---

LEVEL PLAYING FIELD

SPF 20–30: The facial number necessary during the week, if you work in an office.

SPF 40: The amount required on the weekends; the FDA regulates SPF only up to around 40, so there are diminishing returns the higher you go over that number.

---

how you look as the years pass. Proximity to cigarette smoke is a close second. Shielding your face and body from UV light is a guaranteed way to stave off wrinkles. And it's so easy to get sun protection because a plethora of products are formulated with it. You don't even have to do an extra step to ensure basic, everyday coverage because the blocking ingredients are frequently combined with regular moisturizers. If you bypass this part and stop after Step 4, all the hard work you've put in so far on CEAMP will be for naught.

 Ask the Doctor: *I read that the majority of sun damage occurs before the age of eighteen. I'm way past that. Is it too late for me?*

It's never too late. We can always make a difference in our skin's health and the way it feels. Doctors have discovered that patients with precancerous lesions—atypical cells—can alter their skin's function simply by taking off the bad cells and encouraging the body to repair itself. If you mistreated your skin in your youth, you certainly don't want to add to the situation now by continuing to subject your face and body to UV rays. That will only worsen the situation. Don't worry: You can reverse the damage that you might have incurred by adhering to **The Beautiful Skin Workout.**

BUSINESS CASUAL

When you're dressed during the workweek, you get some sun exposure through your clothes, but I wouldn't obsess over it. That's not where the root of your skin issues are going to be. I'm more concerned about safeguarding what's visible on Saturdays and Sundays when you're likely to spend more hours outdoors. Monday through Friday, you just need to apply your SPF to your face and hands—include your chest as well, if you have on a V-neck shirt.

CLOUD COVER

On gray, rainy days, you're still receiving UV exposure. It can even be worse than what you obtain during sunny weather because the clouds trap the light rays. Those then ping back and forth between the ground and the sky. People often end up with bad burns when they're outside in hazy conditions because they don't realize that they're in the presence of so much UV.

Ask the Doctor: *I'm spending Christmas in the Caribbean. Isn't it okay for me to visit a tanning bed a few times beforehand, so that I don't end up roasted on vacation?*

I hear this all the time. There's no such thing as a "base color" when it comes to your skin. It's a ridiculous idea. You're extending your zone of UV exposure by lying in a tanning bed. The way to prevent a burn is by wearing sunblock and staying out of the rays. On your first day at the beach, remain under the umbrella from eleven in the morning until two in the afternoon. Reapply your skin protection every few hours, especially if you're sweating. There are waterproof versions of sunblock, but resistance to water makes a formulation occlusive. You might not opt for those if you're worried they'll clog your pores, especially since you have to reapply the waterproof kind nearly as often as the regular stuff.

BROWNIE POINTS

Sunbathing is never okay. You just can't do it. Still, there are people who like a little color in their skin. *Self-tanning is the only safe method for achieving a dark, deep skin tone.* The tanning ingredient, DHA, reacts with only the most superficial layer of dead cells. It doesn't really penetrate, and it's not a dye. Many products are tinted to allow you to see where to apply them since DHA itself is clear. I'm not a fan of artificial dyes, so I suggest finding a lotion with natural caramel coloring instead, if you're craving an instant bronze.

Even if a self-tanner contains SPF, its UV protection is no greater or longer-lasting than what you'd get from a sunblock. You'll still need to be fastidious about coating yourself with SPF when you're outside. Since dry, flaky skin often ends up streaky after the DHA sets, it's a good idea to exfoliate first from head to toe. This increases the life span of your tan as well since you're removing the cells that are just about to be shed naturally. Conversely, if you scrub the tissue after the tanner has gone to work, you'll quickly make your new hue a memory. You may want to go easy on the body exfoliation, including alpha hydroxy acids, for a few days after you've self-tanned.

Perspiration also causes these items to develop unevenly, so many men and women prefer to smooth their lotion on at night—as opposed to slathering it on right before they hit the beach—and allow it to work while they sleep. The process can take three to four hours, on average, to reach its full effect.

 Ask the Doctor: *Are spray tans safe?*

I certainly wouldn't want to breathe in all those chemicals. I think that's harmful. While I understand people's need for color, going to a self-tanning booth, which mists a large quantity of dye all over your body, can't be good. And we don't know about the long-term effects of inhaling those tiny particles. They were never formulated to be taken internally, so they haven't been rigorously tested for safety when ingested.

COFFEE TALK

If you apply your SPF in the morning, you cannot expect it to protect your skin all day. When the weather is nice and you decide to eat your lunch outside, put on more SPF before exiting the office. Sun preparations last only an hour or two. The sunblock you smoothed on before breakfast will definitely have worn off by noon.

BREAKDOWN LANE

Sunscreens disintegrate faster than sunblocks, so you have to reapply them more often. The new chemical UV blockers (Mexoryl et al.) aren't supposed to dissolve as quickly as the older chemical versions, such as Avobenzone, but the downside is that they're not yet widely available.

EVENING SHADE

You often read that you shouldn't wear your UV protection at night, but that depends on what your UV protection is. Sunblock usually contains zinc, a mineral that's good for skin. If you rubbed that in before bed, you'd actually be doing yourself a favor. However, if you're using sunscreen, then you're adding chemicals that don't really benefit your face and body during the night, so I'd skip it.

Ask the Doctor: *What will erase my stretch marks?*

The entire CEAMP system will help improve the appearance of new or existing stretch marks. Exfoliation, especially with an at-home microdermabrasion scrub, speeds cellular turnover; applying an antiaging cream, even the one you use around your eyes, will give the area the wherewithal to mend itself; moisturization keeps the skin from drying out; and protection helps prevent more tissue breakdown. All these steps will minimize your places of concern. The change may be minor, but you'll definitely see it. When the tissue is healthy, the skin looks better overall.

HARD EVIDENCE

It's one thing for me to tell you how my **Beautiful Skin Workout** can change the texture, quality, and health of your face and body skin. However, as a scientist, I can understand the need for verifiable data to demonstrate that the program truly works. In the next chapter, I present five real-life case studies of men and women who adhered to my regimen. I'll let the results speak for themselves.

Chapter 4

Design Your *Beautiful Skin Workout*

Now that I've explained all the components of my program and what you'll be required to do in order to obtain Creamy skin, I'm sure you're eager to get started. In the Introduction, I asked you to take my Elbow Test to determine your skin type: alligator, leather, sandpaper, rubber, or suede. Knowing the category that best describes your skin texture is the first step in designing your personalized **Beautiful Skin Workout**. I've reiterated the importance of listening to your skin to determine its needs. The main purpose of this guide is to give you tools to understand how skin functions, so that taking care of it will become as natural and easy for you as reciting your ABCs. Then you won't have to follow what someone else is telling you—you'll already know what to do.

Just look around—each person is different. **The Beautiful Skin Workout** enables you to tailor your Cleanse, Exfoliate, Activate, Moisturize, and Protect (CEAMP) program accordingly. **The Beautiful Skin Workout** transforms every kind of skin—alligator, leather, sandpaper, rubber, or suede—but customization will improve your results immensely. To help you personalize your plan, this chapter includes testimonials from five people, each with one of my skin designations. I've outlined the advice I gave, the types of products I suggested, and how the routine can be modified. Additionally, I've noted the number of weeks it took for him or her to reach Creamy skin. After reviewing these real-life examples, I hope you will have everything you need to draw up your own CEAMP plan.

ALLIGATOR

 James, 59, investor

In general, I don't do anything to my skin. I'm probably even more extreme than most guys in terms of taking care of my face. I play a lot of sports, so I'm in the shower all the time, but I haven't used soap to wash my face in years. I either shampoo it or just let the water beat on it, then shave. I don't have a heavy beard, so I don't even need shaving cream.

My complexion is very fair, and I never wore sunblock as a kid. As a result, I've had a number of benign precancerous lesions removed from my face and body. My skin is kind of dry, and I've noticed that I have some dark spots on the backs of my hands, my chest, and my neck. The patches haven't appeared on my face, though.

My wife takes very good care of her skin, and seeing how great she looks is making me think that I need to start doing something as well. I'm not overly worried about it, but I have become more aware.

Intake Assessment

James is a perfect example of someone for whom skin is almost an afterthought. He's busy with work and all his athletic activities; he wasn't going to carve out a large chunk of time for a new grooming regimen. James had brown patches, precancerous lesions, and tough skin. Clearly, he needed a lot, but I couldn't spring it on him all at once. I had to ease him into a routine and let him see for himself how his skin quality improved. If you give people the basics, they eventually embrace a more complete program.

I tiptoed into convincing him to take action. In order to accomplish that goal, I called on my principles of Cosmetic Wellness. **The Beautiful Skin Workout** is an eight-week program that delivers healthy skin, not simply fewer lines and wrinkles. I pointed out his sun damage and potential skin cancers. Even if James weren't concerned with the way he looked, he'd want to safeguard his health.

Doctor's Orders

We started slowly, but I still gave James some recommendations that would deliver beneficial results in a short period of time. I felt that positive reinforcement was likely to convince him to remain committed. James obviously wasn't cleaning his skin properly—he was barely cleaning it at all. If I could have gotten him to switch from shampoo or plain water to a formulation specifically for the face, that would have been fantastic. But some people, usually men, refuse to modify their shower routine. They simply say, "This is the way I do things, and I'm not going to change." Since men don't wear cosmetics, washing is actually not as important for them as it is for women who make up their faces with foundation, powders, and blush. It's fine. I'm trying to help you change your skin, not your personality.

Even though he shaves, James still needed to exfoliate his skin. Shaving is a physical exfoliation, but it's not done all over the face. James had previous skin cancer issues and was complaining about the dark patches on his hands and body. I noticed that the skin along his forehead, near the hairline, was scaly—an indication of potential precancerous lesions. Many men forget about this area when they're applying sunblock to their faces.

I suggested he rub a gentle AHA cream on his nose, hands, and any other UV-exposed areas he hadn't immediately gone over with the razor. I added a pigment-blocking formula to his arsenal of products, as well as sun protection, and had him try this regimen for two weeks, twice a day.

Routine Maintenance

After fourteen days, James had noticed some improvement in his skin's texture and tone and returned to my office ready to do more for his face and hands. At this stage, I handed him a nutrient-rich vitamin C booster spray. Antioxidants help skin heal itself, and we know James has sun damage. I also suggested an antiaging eye cream and a toning aftershave, so that he could balance his skin, even if he wasn't washing it.

Final Analysis

James took more than eight weeks to get to Creamy skin, but he was firmly in suede territory by the end of the two months. When you're attempting to convince someone who's never paid much attention to his skin to shift his mind-set and start looking after his face, it can be a long process. I'm not saying it can't be done, but probably not at the rate you initially hoped for. James understood that exfoliation leads to skin rejuvenation. Making that connection was a vital component of adherence to **The Beautiful Skin Workout**.

James didn't lose all the discoloration on the backs of his hands. This doesn't mean that he was a failure at following **The Beautiful Skin Workout**. Some brown spots are so deep that they must be zapped with a laser in order to be totally erased. But pigment-reducing creams combined with this routine can make those areas much lighter, softer, and smoother. By prepping the tissue in this manner, you'll recover more quickly from any physician-administered procedure you may undergo later.

HEAD GAMES

Men who have receding hairlines or bald patches receive a lot of sun on those areas, so it's extremely important for them to put sunscreen on their foreheads and bare skin. Ears are another potential danger zone. Males are more likely than females to report skin cancers on the tops of their ears, because hair is a natural protectant. Without it, skin is much more prone to developing cancer. It's a real problem for men. They need to shield their heads with a hat and sunblock. You can, and should, CEAMP those vulnerable places as well.

Ask the Doctor: *If I'm not going to do all five steps, is there a chance for my skin?*

There are people who believe that five is too many, and they're simply not going to do all of them. It's not *horrible* if a man enters the shower and uses bar soap on his face. If you refuse to apply antioxidants, all hope is not lost. It's not great, but we're not living in a perfect world.

LEATHER

Suzanne, 61, fashion executive

I have extremely fair skin naturally. Despite that, I would get so dark in the summertime that my friends would say that I looked Indian. I just lived in the sun and used to coat myself in iodine and baby oil, if you can believe it. When I was growing up, people didn't know that UV light was dangerous.

Thanks to all of that unrepentant tanning and my fair complexion, I knew that I would have skin issues eventually. I now get full-body mole checks at least twice a year. On my arm, I've had one spot removed, which turned out to be a precancerous lesion. Another place on my neck actually was a basal cell carcinoma. Nothing on my face has required surgery, but I do have one crusty sunspot that doesn't seem to go away. And the texture on my cheeks, where I had received so much sun, is thicker and heavier than other areas of my face. Even though my facial tissue is thin, it's still leathery and dull.

I've used all the upscale skin-care products on the market. I've gone back and forth between different brands but never settled on anything. Of course we're all concerned about lines. I'd love to get rid of my wrinkles. I'm the only one among my friends who hasn't had plastic surgery. I'm not morally opposed to it; I'm just not into the extreme look so many women have these days. I want to grow old gracefully, but I want to do it with good skin.

Intake Assessment

A person such as Suzanne will benefit from regulating her skin function via a fixed program. Consistently exfoliating will help get rid of any precancerous cells on her face and body, particularly important for a person such as Suzanne who's a prime candidate for skin cancer.

Doctor's Orders

I started Suzanne on the basic five steps. Since she was a bit of a product junkie, this was pretty easy. I also had her throw out all the extra items in her bathroom. That took a little more convincing. Since her thin skin was slightly sensitive, despite being leathery, I had Suzanne exfoliate with a gentle AHA lotion, in addition to applying an antioxidant serum and a pigment lightener. She was already conscious about loading up on SPF, so I didn't need to give her my usual talk. After four weeks, we added antiaging creams to the mix, and she began polishing her face weekly with a light honey almond scrub.

Final Analysis

At eight weeks, Suzanne had suede skin. The feel and appearance of her complexion were vastly improved. The discolored patches had faded to almost nothing. With continued care, she can expect to be in the Creamy category. To speed up her skin's renewal process, Suzanne also began occasional in-office treatments, such as microdermabrasion combined with nonablative laser and intense pulsed light sessions (more about those in Chapter 5).

Suzanne had been jumping around from skin-care plan to skin-care plan, but I'm not worried about her sticking to this one. Her primary concern is health. I can tell that by the way she's been regularly evaluating herself for moles. Exfoliating her face and body has become just one more aspect of cancer prevention for Suzanne. Even texture and reduced lines are a welcome bonus.

SANDPAPER

 Emily, 27, nonprofit executive

I've never been a smoker or sunbather. I don't have much, if any, sun damage, nor do I have problems with wrinkles. That's the good news. The flip side is that I have horrible cystic acne on my cheeks. It comes and goes, but that area of my face is pretty much always red. The strange thing is that my complexion isn't really oily; if anything, it's dry and scabby. And it really, really hurts. My skin's so sensitive to the products I apply to treat the acne that I can't use one for too long. Of course, nothing seems to work anyway.

I can't say that I have a particular skin-care regimen. I try to cleanse with the right things and to moisturize, but my experiences have shown me that the more I do, the worse my face gets. I'm pretty embarrassed and frustrated, and at the same time I feel as though there's no solution. My skin has been like this since puberty, and I think it's just something that I'm going to have to live with for the rest of my life.

Intake Assessment

Emily's skin was extremely sensitive; you could tell just by looking at her face that it was painful. I often see the same thing with patients suffering from rosacea, eczema, psoriasis, or excessive flaking. It's hard to get these types of skin on a standardized program. The tissue is so reactive to everything with which it comes in contact that a little bit of stress or a change in routine can turn it blotchy and red, and patients whose skin is this quick to flare are generally reluctant to do anything to it for fear of triggering a negative outcome.

I noticed something else when I met Emily for the first time. She had some facial hair in areas you wouldn't expect to see on someone her age, and she mentioned her irregular periods. This information, combined with the facial cysts, made me think that Emily might have some other health issues. I sent her to an endocrinologist, who confirmed my suspicions: Emily had polycystic ovary disorder, a hormonal imbalance. The medicine she started taking for her condition regulated her hormone levels, helping clear her skin, but we still needed to take care of the faint acne scars that had developed and reduce her skin's sensitivity.

Perhaps more than any other group, the reactive sandpaper varieties need to be attuned to their skin and not get disheartened if breakouts appear all of a sudden. That's going to happen. If you fall into this category, take a deep breath, tweak what you're doing, and continue on. The causes may even be factors that you can't control, like humidity, which challenges your skin. However, you—and Emily—can still reach the Creamy designation.

Doctor's Orders

I usually start a reactive-skinned patient on **The Beautiful Skin Workout** slowly: cleanser, toner, moisturizer, and sunblock. I don't want him or her to exfoliate right away; just these four initial things help heal the skin. In many ways, achieving Creamy skin is a joint process between patient and doctor. I can observe a women's face when she's in my examining room, but once she returns home, I count on her to keep track of the way she's responding to each topical we introduce. That's the way we ascertain which products are having a beneficial effect. After we're sure that these four basic components aren't causing any problems (this takes about one week), I have the person apply a mild AHA cream every other day and slowly increase to twice-daily use over the next six weeks.

Pace Yourself

If you're sensitive, there might be a formulation, even if it's free of fragrances and dyes and is allergy tested, that simply does not agree with your complexion. I don't ask these patients to begin too many things at once, as then we won't be able to tell what's causing an adverse response. If a woman's skin begins to erupt, she usually wants to stop everything she's on. We end up backtracking and losing time. This happens quite a bit, actually, and not

---

NATURAL PROGRESSION

Men and women with reactive skin often have problems all over their bodies, not just on their faces. They could CEAMP their arms, legs, and elbows. The same positive improvements they see in their complexions will be repeated on the areas beneath the chin.

---

just with sensitive skin. People sprint forward and then have a setback.

Final Analysis

As I said, when I meet patients with delicate complexions, I hold off on in-office microdermabrasion because I like to prep the skin for a week or two with the proper care. However, I'm able to modulate the way I work this exfoliation machine. Emily's skin was red, but also dry and patchy. If I performed microdermabrasion, I could give Emily an immediate textural improvement, which would have taken three weeks to achieve with skin care alone, so I exfoliated her face on day one. By following the CEAMP plan for the next eight weeks, Emily cleared up the redness and got rid of the scars. She has maybe two left now, but they are so faint that I don't think even she notices them.

If the ruddiness hadn't disappeared on its own, the next step would have been laser treatments to eradicate the blood vessels that had formed. By the time we'd be ready to start those, the quality of the facial tissue would be vastly improved.

RUBBER

 Anne, 52, trial attorney

One day, I glanced in the mirror and thought, Oh my gosh, I look like my mother. In my field, appearing healthy and vibrant, as opposed to tired and haggard, gives a woman an

edge in terms of believability. I'm not saying that I want to pass for a twenty-one-year-old, but I'm very uncomfortable and self-conscious about my appearance right now. My skin just doesn't look good. I don't get breakouts, but there's something about my face's tone—I can't describe it—that's preventing it from being attractive.

I grew up in a family in which everyone used soap to wash his or her face. My mother never wore makeup. I didn't apply moisturizer or sunscreen, but my skin was always relatively clear. It wasn't until I hit forty that things went downhill—and fast. I should probably admit that I sleep with my foundation and eye shadow on. I don't want my husband to see me without them because my bare face looks awful. My eyes don't seem bright, and the texture is simply not okay.

When I prepare to go to court, I become obsessed about the way I look. I'll put on four different suits, figuring out which one makes my face more striking. I'm spending all this time trying to ensure that I'm presenting the best image. I feel that I appear older than I am.

Intake Assessment

There are some who argue that wanting to be beautiful is a sign of superficiality. While I agree that one should never become so consumed with her appearance that it takes over her life, I've witnessed firsthand the dramatic impact a woman's appearance can have on her self-esteem and outlook. Anne is a perfect example. She's a smart, funny, warm person, and I felt sorry that she was so down. At the same time, I was incredibly hopeful and optimistic because a few small modifications to her skin-care routine (or rather, creating one, since she kept going back to soap and water) would have a startling impact on Anne's face and on her image of herself.

Doctor's Orders

I couldn't believe that Anne was sleeping in her makeup! Convincing her to wash her face at night with a gentle cleanser—and leave it bare—would have made Anne's skin so much better that I probably could have just stopped there. Anne also had sunspots on her face and legs, as well as some fine lines. She was right, though: Texture was the main issue.

By the time Anne entered my office, she had almost reached her wit's end. She was desperate for a solution to her complexion woes and enthusiastically adopted all five CEAMP steps. Anne also promised not to reapply her foundation before bed. To combat the dark patches that had formed on her face and body, I gave her a pigment-reducing cream to slather on twice daily. Exfoliation was the most efficient method for increasing the radiance in her complexion. With her twenty-four-hour-a-day cosmetics habit, Anne certainly wasn't allowing her cells much of a chance to slough off on their own. We needed to fire up the cellular manufacturing system with AHAs morning and night.

Final Analysis

Anne's results were beyond her wildest dreams. It wasn't just that she got to Creamy skin in five weeks. She started leaving the house, during the day, without makeup.

She told me that her children couldn't believe it. They had literally never seen their mother's skin devoid of some sort of cosmetic. She appears healthy and glowing and says that her work is going much better as well. Now that she's not wasting hours deciding on her outfit, she can focus her energy on her caseload.

Anne wanted to take things even farther. Once she saw an improvement in her face's firmness and texture, she was encouraged to get rid of her deep frown lines. Eventually, she did submit to a few hyaluronic acid injections. Sometimes people have major wrinkles—they need a skin filler. Not every problem is cured with topical creams, but they can do an awful lot. Undergoing surgical procedures without tending to the tissue in advance just doesn't make sense.

SUEDE

Margaret, 34, cosmetics developer

Even though I work in the beauty business, I've never really paid any mind to my skin. My job involves makeup, not skin care, so I'm not exposed to all the latest age-reversing creams and wrinkle-erasing serums. I've been washing my face with a "beauty bar" since I was practically an infant. I do apply moisturizer from head to toe, so my skin is soft. Breakouts have never been a problem for me, so overall I was feeling that my skin was in pretty good shape.

I'd say that the one bad habit I have is lying out. Describing myself as a sun worshipper doesn't even begin to cover it. Some people are addicted to cigarettes or coffee; for me, it's the feeling of the rays beating down on my skin. I love it, and my parents are the same way. They previously used reflectors and got very, very dark. In the winter, I go to a tanning bed once a week, just to keep up my color, and I always vacation in sunny places, like the Caribbean. I never wore sunscreen—I was a baby oil girl who slowly shifted into SPF 4 and 6 and is now smoothing on SPF 8 or 10.

Despite always basking in the sun, it wasn't until I hit thirty that I developed lines on my face. But once the crow's feet came, they were bad. My eye area is the only part of my face that's showing signs of aging. I'm starting to notice some dark spots on my chest, but my complexion is fine. I've used every eye cream on the market since I'm able to get samples through work. Nothing has erased the wrinkles. Maybe I'm not sticking with them long enough, but when I try something and it's not making a difference, I move on. I'm not ready for injections; I want a topical solution.

Intake Assessment

As hard as it is to believe, with all the UV exposure she's had, Margaret's skin actually looked decent. She's not a smoker, and the rest of her lifestyle is pretty healthy. The crow's feet were visible, but the rest of her face was in okay shape—for now. Her skin wasn't sensitive, so she jumped right into **The Beautiful Skin Workout**.

Doctor's Orders

The lines around her eyes are just the first indication of what's to come if Margaret doesn't begin caring for her

skin and wearing protection year-round. And by protection, I don't mean SPF 10, which is practically useless. She needs SPF 40, at the minimum. The sunbathing has got to stop. At the very least, she must halt the tanning bed sessions. Those machines are the worst; they assault your skin with pure UVA rays—the very ones that rip into collagen and destroy the fibers holding the tissue up.

It's often a significant adjustment for someone who's never followed a multipart skin-care plan to remain faithful to each component day and night. I really commend Margaret for keeping at it. She initially asked for only a good eye product, but I explained to her that just as you can't spot-tone a single section of your body, like saddle-

EASY DOES IT

When a patient is new to eye products, I advise her to start slowly. The eye tissue needs the extra nutrients in a specialized item, but you don't want to rush into it. If you develop sensitivity issues due to your undereye product, part of the problem may be that you're applying it right before going to bed. When you lie back on the pillow, your body heat can cause the formula to melt and seep into your lashes. Evaluate a potential fragrance-free, allergy-tested eye cream or serum by dabbing it on right above your cheekbones during your evening CEAMP ritual. If you don't have a reaction the next day, apply it to the upper lid, staying close to the orbital bone to avoid getting the ingredients in your eye. The final step is tracing the cream along the under-eye socket as well.

bag thighs, you need to attend to all of your skin if you want your crow's feet to disappear. When the entire system is healthy, it reflects well on the individual parts. With that in mind, Margaret adopted the five steps twice daily—including eye cream.

Final Analysis

Margaret reached Creamy skin in three weeks. And she began experimenting with self-tanner. That was huge for her. Margaret admits that she still wants to broil under the sun. She hasn't had a personality transplant, after all.

What will keep her on the program is the enhancement in her skin. Now that she's aware of how it functions, she realizes that there's a lot more where those crow's feet came from. She's going to be proactive about keeping the indicators of aging at bay. Exfoliating and layering on antioxidants helps repair some of the damage lurking underneath the surface. Guarding her skin will prevent new wrinkles from cropping up.

Ask the Doctor: *On your program, will my skin worsen before it gets better, especially if I have acne?*

Outbreaks can happen occasionally—don't become discouraged. Bringing your skin into balance takes time. When you begin an exercise program, you may develop sore muscles as your body adapts to the new routine. Your skin behaves similarly. You might have to back off the CEAMP routine a little, especially the exfoliant step, to help clear your skin if it suddenly acts up.

THE $64,000 QUESTION: HOW LONG DOES THE BEAUTIFUL SKIN WORKOUT TAKE?

You need to remain allegiant to the program I've laid out for you. The amount of time required for you to reach Creamy skin will depend on how far you have to go. Suede

---

CHARTING IT OUT

 If you adhere to **The Beautiful Skin Workout**, the following time periods should be in the ballpark of when you'll reach Creamy skin:

 Alligator: six to eight weeks

 Leather: six to eight weeks

 Rubber: four to six weeks

 Sandpaper: two to four weeks

 Suede: two to four weeks

---

types will reach their goal at a much more rapid pace than their alligator friends. Applying topical skin care is a lot like dressing for winter: the more layers, the better. Don't hesitate to smooth an antioxidant-rich vitamin C serum over a pigment-reducing kojic acid cream over an acne-erasing salicylic acid compound. You'll note your skin improving way before a person who simply slaps on moisturizer.

TAKE IT EASY

Who's perfect? No one I know. Ideally, there'd be enough hours in the day for us to exercise, eat right, take moments for ourselves, de-stress, and spend time with our friends and families. I myself have never had a day even close to this. The principles of **The Beautiful Skin Workout,** consistency and healthy habits, can still apply. Like an athlete, you need to train regularly to meet your goals. But don't beat yourself up if you slip. Creamy skin is something that you'll maintain forever, not simply a few months. Once you've achieved it, don't worry that you'll undo all your progress in one day.

RETURN INVESTMENT

The most important thing to keep in mind is that whatever your skin looks like after eight weeks, it hasn't reached a plateau. The condition of your face and body is only going to get better. I have patients who began my program two years ago. When I see them now, their skin appears even smoother and more radiant, as hard to believe as that may sound. Their skin is *younger* today than it was two years ago. It's Cosmetic Wellness. The results surprise me, too, even though I see them all the time. **The Beautiful Skin Workout** is a continuous, lifelong routine. You don't cycle on and off of it. The rewards are numerous, including the fact that you're not going to age as quickly as those who aren't on the program.

You might begin by applying **The Beautiful Skin Workout** strictly to your face. But after you've seen how great your complexion has become I hope you'll expand your CEAMP plan to the rest of your body. That's smart behavior. All of your skin, from head to heel, needs **The Beautiful Skin Workout** to be healthy and glowing. CEAMPing will become so fast and easy that anything less just won't feel right.

MOVING ON

If you have acne scarring, sagging skin, or another, more serious skin concern, CEAMP may not be the be-all and end-all for you. What I'm hoping is that **The Beautiful Skin Workout** can make a difference in your appearance. I am sure of its beneficial effects. You will look better. You may not look as good as you want, though. In the final chapter, I'll explain some of the in-office options for treating issues that **The Beautiful Skin Workout**, and topical skin care in general, is unable to remedy completely.

Chapter 5

The Future of Skin

This is an exciting time in cosmetic surgery. There have been incredible innovations and pioneering advances in antiaging techniques, including radiofrequency, lasers, and other light-based initiatives. Skin rejuvenation is truly in its golden age. There are targeted, effective solutions out there for almost every skin concern: rosacea, varicose veins, brown spots, cystic acne, and wrinkles, to name just a few. With proper guidance, a person can resolve almost anything that's plaguing her face or body.

I've traveled the globe, lecturing in France, Italy, Scotland, Cyprus, Russia, and China. The desire for powerful antiaging measures and proven ways to turn back the clock isn't simply a U.S. phenomenon. Every place I visit, colleagues want to discuss the latest discoveries in plastic surgery and the developments in skin care. We now know that we can stimulate our bodies, at the deepest cellular level, to function as they're supposed to naturally. As we age, those internal mechanisms slow down, but new scientific discoveries are showing us how to override our inherent tendencies. Today we can confidently promise our patients—and, more important, deliver—Creamy, youthful skin.

ACCEPT NO SUBSTITUTES

The information in this chapter is not intended to replace CEAMPing. The procedures I'll describe should be considered in conjunction with your established skin-care routine. For people who have the time and money, these treatments will help speed the path to Creamy skin. For issues that CEAMP cannot remedy, such as scarring or deep pigmentation, some of these steps may be the only fix. No matter what you decide, you'll heal much, much faster if you've been properly tending to your skin in advance of heading to your physician's office.

TURN ON THE LIGHTS

The number of wavelengths of energy is infinite. Doctors have been able to harness certain spectrums to achieve a variety of skin rejuvenation and repair goals. There's always a plus and a minus in any procedure, and I'm not willing to chance scarring except in the most extreme cases. However, the bulk of the light-based technologies are safe, and their negative occurrence rate is extremely low. I recommend those with confidence to my patients.

The modalities used for cosmetic purposes are grouped into the following categories:

Ablative lasers: Ablation means the removal of tissue. Ablative lasers, such as the CO_2 or Erbium, essentially vaporize the epidermis, the top layer of skin, leaving a person's face raw and red for several weeks. On the positive side, when the tissue finally regenerates, it's often firmer and smoother than it was previously, with fewer wrinkles. However, there's a possibility that during the healing process, you might experience an alteration in your melanin, either developing too much or too little. I'm not a big proponent of this type of resurfacing, both because of its considerable recovery period and its occasional tendency to create discoloration and scarring. What's the point of having a lineless face if you have to cover it with foundation every time you go outside? When you are considering this protocol, you'll need to weigh its beauty benefits against its pigmentation risks. The patches you end up with could be worse than the wrinkle you had.

Nonablative lasers: All lasers use thermal energy, but nonablative beams bypass the visible tissue and head straight to the dermis. This stimulates collagen growth. The surface of the skin remains relatively unaffected by a nonablative session, so it's rare for a patient's face to be blotchy or inflamed afterward. Dermal tissue recoils as it's heated, making the complexion tighter right away; you could see an immediate, positive skin change. However, while one course of an ablative laser does bring results, four to six monthly nonablative treatments are typically needed for noticeable long-term gains. Repeating a nonablative procedure creates more collagen and has a cumulative effect.

Fractional resurfacing: Ablative and nonablative lasers have been around for some time. Now there is a new category: fractionated lasers. Some of the best known of this group are the Fraxel, ActiveFX, and Lux 1540. Researchers have discovered that if you don't remove the entire top layer of skin, as you do with an ablative device, and instead leave small, untouched spaces, you get a faster improvement than with a nonablative laser but without the ablative's dangers.

Fractionated lasers make tiny pinpricks in the skin. The holes are invisible to the naked eye, but the tissue that's been zapped does flake off. Patients often report visible shedding for a couple of days postprocedure. The treatment's thermal energy rebuilds collagen. It's a little more aggressive than the nonablative machines, so a doctor can do more in a single session. While fewer visits are necessary, compared to nonablatives, you may still need to go more than once to achieve your optimal outcome.

My busy patients don't want any downtime—a few days of puffiness or scaling are a turn-off. I get such good results from stacking therapies like Nd:YAG laser and IPL, without even the smallest bit of inflammation. Few patients are requesting fractional resurfacing. Improvements in this technology should lessen those negative side effects, however, and amplify the positives.

Intense pulsed light (IPL): A laser emits one single beam, which is a specific wavelength. That energy setting is dependent on the result the physician wants, such as collagen formation. IPL is a diffuse shot of light, traveling at different wavelengths simultaneously. Its energy isn't as concentrated as that from a laser, nor is it as powerful. For these reasons, it may take several IPL sessions to reach the same point as one or two laser visits. However, the treatment is much gentler on the skin than laser. It's a trade-off worth discussing with your physician before you commit to a protocol.

Light-emitting diodes (LEDs): LEDs may be the next step in light-based skin therapy. We know that light has a thermal effect, and it's the foundation upon which lasers—ablative and non—work. Scientists have proved that high temperatures encourage skin mending and collagen growth. Now researchers are wondering if light, not heat, energy could change the way tissue works.

That's the premise of LEDs. A patient sits in front of a panel of tiny blinking bulbs sometimes for as little as a minute. Repeated exposure in the areas subjected to the flashing stimulates collagen formation. LEDs generate an extremely small dose of power, so they seem to involve very little risk. Medical advances may even lead to a safe low-level light device for home use. LEDs deliver minor restorations over long blocks of time, but the concept of reduced amounts of light energy bundled in a way that, without pain or discomfort, gives therapeutic benefits is universally appealing. As a result, in the next year or two, we'll see enhancements in this field.

Ask the Doctor: Is the light from a laser or similar device the same as what the sun puts out?

No, not at all. You don't have to worry that by submitting to IPL, LEDs, or a laser that you're going to end up looking older instead of younger. Light arrives in many different wavelengths. On the UV spectrum, the rays that you need to be concerned with are UVA and UVB. Red, blue, infrared, and other varieties in the new light-based technologies aren't going to destroy your existing collagen or ramp up the rate at which you're aging.

WHERE DO WE GO FROM HERE?

No one wants to walk around oozing and raw, the way ablative patients have to. However, it's difficult to argue with the dramatic benefits the process delivers after one session. The question is: How can we get ablative results using nonablative technology? I became frustrated with the limitations of each modality available, so I put them together and found that I could make the whole greater than the sum of its parts. Eventually we'll have single devices, which join separate therapies such as laser, IPL, and radiofrequency in one handpiece.

Even though the treatment frequency necessary with nonablative or fractional resurfacing isn't huge, technological advancements will undoubtedly help reduce those numbers. Already doctors have been tweaking these systems, modifying thermal pulses or duration or developing new skin-cooling modalities. Now the steps are being refined, giving physicians more control over the process. The goal of medical innovation continues to be greater efficacy with less skin trauma.

Ask the Doctor: *My skin tone is very deep naturally. Are light-based therapies for me?*

Scientific knowledge in this area has really improved over the past few years. Today, with precautions and extra measures, IPL and lasers are safe for people of all ethnicities. Often the devices' energy levels must be reduced or the wavelength manipulated, so it may take more visits to score satisfactory results. If this lessens the risk associated with these types of procedures, it's a small trade-off.

IT'S THE PITS

The problem: Acne scarring

The prescription: Nonablative lasers (like the CoolTouch, Polaris, or Smoothbeam) or fractional resurfacing lasers

The promise: These wavelengths stimulate collagen production, building up a skin depression from underneath.

The process: The lasers' heat melts collagen slightly, triggering the body to manufacture even more of the fibers as replacements. Generally, it takes six monthly nonablative visits or two to three fractional resurfacing sessions to plump a scar. One bonus side effect of both? They reduce the appearance of wrinkles and improve skin texture in almost everyone, even those without scars.

The prediction: While existing options are effective at minimizing acne marks, these lasers may have to be employed repeatedly over long periods if the depression is extremely profound. As the science guiding the development of nonablative and fractionated equipment improves, those tools will become powerful enough to repair deep pits in just a few sessions.

Reality Show

Simon, 24, graduate student

I had some mild acne scars, which I wanted to get rid of. I wasn't familiar with the various things a doctor could do to even the skin's texture and color. Dr. Copeland told me about the success she'd had on her patients using a nonablative laser, which fills in the depressions.

I went for four sessions. Dr. Copeland suggested six, but I've been so busy with school that I haven't been able to get back to her office. The treatment wasn't painful at all. It felt more like a mild bee sting. It's also pretty short—about a minute or two. I'm Asian, and I was a little wary about how my skin would react to the laser. It ended up not being a problem.

I'd say my complexion used to be a six, on a scale of one to ten. Now it's an eight and a half. I'm happy with it overall. I achieved the results I wanted.

RED, RED WHINE

The problem: Broken capillaries, dilated blood vessels, and spider veins

The prescription: IPL or lasers, like the Pulsed Dye or Nd:YAG

The promise: Light energy that homes in on ruddy pigment, erasing red areas on the face and body.

The process: When using a laser, a doctor does one pass, or several, over sections with persistent redness. The wavelength recognizes only high concentrations of pigment in the visible capillaries. Once heated, those vessels shrivel and disappear. In most cases, one to two laser sessions spaced over four to six weeks are necessary to reach complete clearance. Postprocedure, skin may be slightly irritated for a few days.

IPL is milder than lasers but requires multiple courses—usually four to six. The nice thing about an IPL treatment is that it gives you the added benefit of tissue tightening.

The prediction: For very prominent redness, such as the veins around the nose, a laser is the best removal option. IPL isn't always strong enough to complete the job. However, since most people prefer to go straight back to work after a medical visit, researchers are finding ways to mesh the low adverse reaction rate of IPL with lasers' potency.

Ask the Doctor: *Isn't it easier to have red or brown spots burned off?*

The process you're referring to is called cauterization. It's an older method of removing pigmented lesions. Freezing is another. These techniques are more traumatic to skin than a laser. They also have a larger chance of creating a scar. In everything we do, our goal is to keep tissue injury to a minimum. We're able to meet that standard when using a laser; we can't guarantee the same results with cauterization or freezing.

TUNNEL VISION

The problem: Varicose veins

The prescription: Laser fiber-based machines, like the EndoVenous Laser Treatment (EVLT)

The promise: Instead of cutting out the offending vein, doctors insert a laser fiber into the vessel and destroy it with heat.

The process: Until very recently, the only procedure for getting rid of varicose veins was referred to as stripping. A surgeon created an incision at the top and bottom of the vessel and then pulled it out. Now we make a single tiny cut to thread the laser—that's it. Thermal energy warms water in the vein wall, shrinking the vein, which the body absorbs. It only takes one session. Recovery time is minimal, especially compared to the weeks usually required to heal from stripping.

The prediction: Currently, some of the largest varicose veins can't be eliminated with fibers, but soon we should be able to use these lasers on vessels of all sizes and this method will become the standard.

PATCH WORK

The problem: Brown spots

The prescription: A laser, such as the Pulsed Dye or Nd:YAG

The promise: These devices dissolve areas of discrete pigment.

The process: When it comes to targeting individual spots on the face, neck, and hands, lasers are the number one choice of many doctors. One shot often breaks up a brown mark completely. A scab, which typically lasts about a week, forms over each place that's been zapped. Once the small crust falls off, the area may be a little red, but that fades over the next several weeks. It's possible that the dark spots will come back. However, diligent application of sunblock and pigment lighteners will help reduce the speed at which they return.

The prediction: We're already observing that people are taking better care of their skin and wearing SPF. That trend is growing, which will mean fewer and lighter brown patches and allow patients to hold off on the more aggressive remedies for excess pigment. My signature treatment is a combination of microdermabrasion, Nd:YAG laser, IPL, and LEDs, which encourages cell turnover and collagen stimulation without downtime. I've discovered that four to six sessions of this mix can also decrease brown spots. As more physicians adopt an integrated method for skin rejuvenation, it will become a solution for erasing accumulated pigment, especially on those patients who don't want any scabbing.

BREAKOUT BREAKDOWN

The problem: Cystic acne

The prescription: Photodynamic therapy (PDT)

The promise: By joining light energy and aminolevulinic acid (ALA), doctors can shrink oil-producing glands.

The process: Physicians paint the skin with clear ALA, a topical photosensitizer, wait for it to sink in, then hit it with light. The drug gathers in areas of clumped cells, like acne or precancerous lesions, creating a target for the beam. A patient typically needs several monthly PDT sessions to minimize acne, as well as an annual follow-up to ensure that skin stays crystal clear. One drawback is that ALA makes the tissue incredibly reactive (especially to the sun), for at least twenty-four hours posttreatment. Sometimes a person may experience a couple of days of swelling or redness. PDT certainly isn't something you'd want to do right before you're attending an important event.

The prediction: As I've said regarding doctor-administered procedures, a treatment with no downtime and a high level of efficacy is one of the holy grails in the antiaging field. We'd like to lessen the sensitivity factor of PDT so that it becomes more palatable to a wider range of men and women.

The skin needs a couple of hours to absorb ALA. That means a couple of hours of sitting in the physician's office waiting for the process to begin or applying the day before treatment. Developing light-sensitive medications with a quicker onset than ALA will be the next step in ameliorating this option.

GET INTO THE GROOVE

The problem: Deep lines

The prescription: Injectables like hyaluronic acid, poly-L-lactic acid, calcium hydroxylapatite, or fat

The promise: These fillers plump deeper crevices and wrinkles (which topical creams alone are unable to erase), in the face and hands.

The process: Using a syringe, a physician lays down one of these products under skin depressions. Hyaluronic acid–based fillers, like Restylane, Hylaform, and Juvaderm, typically last longer than collagen, which has a life span of three to four months, and give a more natural appearance.

Poly-L-lactic acid, available cosmetically under the name Sculptra, is made of the same material as dissolvable sutures. It's an interesting product because while Poly-L-lactic acid itself fills, its presence also motivates the body to produce collagen encasing the substance, similar to seeding a pearl. The body slowly digests the stimulus and only the new collagen remains. Two to four applications spaced over six-week intervals are normally needed to get poly-L-lactic acid's full effect. The fresh fibers are subject to the same breakdown process as other body collagen and, therefore, last about two years. Poly-L-lactic acid is best for treating the overall facial wasting that occurs with age due to loss of fat and other supporting tissue. It's not a good choice for volumizing the lips.

Calcium hydroxylapatite (commonly known as Radiesse) is firmer than hyaluronic or poly-L-lactic acid, so it's a frequent fix for deep, deep grooves and to enhance bony contours, such as the cheeks or chin. The ingredient can remain intact almost twenty-four months. Because of calcium hydroxylapatite's viscosity, I wouldn't add it to the lip area. Doctors are also shaping noses with calcium hydroxylapatite, injecting it on one side of the bridge if the nose is crooked or along the top to disguise a bump.

Fat harvested from a patient's body (usually the stomach or buttocks) and returned to the face has the least chance of triggering an adverse reaction. A large portion of fat is permanent, but to ensure that result, a doctor has to add extra. Recipients walk around for a couple of days with swollen faces, which they often attribute to a "dental procedure." Unused fat can be frozen for six months and injected later if a person desires more fullness.

The characteristic side effects from any of these plumpers are temporary bruising and slight puffiness. Neither persists more than a few days. Sometimes the products may form lumps under the skin, but those subside gradually with massage.

The prediction: You might think that the next logical progression would be to develop an injectable with permanence. Actually, that's not such a great idea. Our bodies are changing all the time. If you add something that's static, it may look natural at first but over decades become steadily more apparent. The main issue with permanent fillers is once you get them in, you can't take them back out. The ideal would be an injectable that lasts two to four years, and we'll have one soon.

BUYER BEWARE

Injection techniques can vary. It's the art and science of what I do, and it's important to choose your doctor wisely. I suggest finding a physician with plenty of experience using these products.

We'll also see more fillers that work to stimulate the body's existing tissue. Poly-L-lactic acid is a good example of the first wave of this technology. This type of product is directed at the cells themselves, engaging them in the antiaging process, instead of letting them sit passively on the sidelines. The results from this form of injectable last longer than the usual suspects—collagen and hyaluronic acid—but still aren't forever.

We're already mimicking some of the skin-relaxing consequences of Botox with topical creams. I'm certain that we'll also create topicals able to inflate the skin selectively. Hyaluronic acid particles are very large, but if they were compressed, they could absorb into lines and expand from underneath.

 Ask the Doctor: *What is Meso-Botox?*

Mesotherapy uses very small, short needles to deliver medicine into the juncture between the dermis and epidermis; it doesn't reach the underlying muscle. The procedure permits doctors to place drugs in targeted sections, rather than asking a patient to take the medicine systemically and hope that it travels to the areas they want. Certain mesotherapy drug combinations allow physicians to help speed the metabolism of fat cells, for example, or reconfigure cellulite formation.

Meso-Botox is a new form of mesotherapy in which very dilute amounts of Botox are injected into the top layer of skin. I find it's particularly effective at reducing crepiness in the neck and relaxing small vertical lines above the mouth. If Botox is injected directly into the muscle above the Cupid's bow, it often causes mouth droop since the muscle over the lip is temporarily paralyzed. In my experience, the effects of Meso-Botox are good for a few months.

SLACKING OFF

The problem: Sagging body skin

The prescription: Radiofrequency devices, like Thermage, and infrared versions, such as Titan

The promise: These energy wavelengths have already been shown to tighten lax facial skin. We've discovered that they do the same thing below the neck.

The process: Many doctors, myself included, now remedy wobbly upper arms, drooping thighs, and postpartum stomachs with either radiofrequency or infrared, which target deeper tissue than lasers. The first generation of Thermage was painful, and patients often complained that the outcome wasn't worth it. However, Thermage handpieces have been redesigned and the recommended energy settings updated. Reports of patient displeasure have dropped, although the procedure is still uncomfortable. Topical anesthetics combined with a mild analgesic are usually sufficient at overcoming this drawback. The good news is that it generally takes only a single one-hour visit, and initially you see some improvement, which continues for the next three to six months. The benefits remain about eighteen months. Infrared instruments such as the Titan, on the other hand, require repeat visits—often three—but the process itself is not painful.

The prediction: Quite a few tools that combine these two modalities are coming out. Ideally, they'll produce even more skin constriction, although obviously not to the same extent as surgery. As there is no recovery period with these initiatives, I see them becoming more mainstream and more accessible. People will begin to regard them as simply a part of routine antiaging maintenance.

Ask the Doctor: *If I have Thermage done on my upper arms, will the results be as good as if I'd had plastic surgery?*

Measures such as Thermage are for people who don't want to undergo an invasive treatment but still desire taut tissue. Skin care isn't going to give you the same lift as Thermage; Thermage won't deliver an outcome akin to surgery. The improvements of each option are on different levels. If you start taking care of your skin early using **The Beautiful Skin Workout**, however, you may not need to go to extremes later.

Reality Show

Audrey, 45, merchandise planner

I had lost a lot of weight, so my skin was loose and hanging. My underarms, in particular, were like batwings. I looked like Jabba the Hut. I had to buy blouses two sizes larger to fit my arms. I just wanted to chop them off.

Dr. Copeland convinced me to try a combination of liposuction and Thermage on my underarms because of the scarring that would occur with surgery. As she pointed out, I could always go back later and cut out the skin if I wasn't happy with the combo treatment.

Well, the results were nothing short of a miracle. I can fit in my tops, and there are no visible marks. I can't say enough about it. Dr. Copeland said that I'd get about a 30 percent lift in the skin after the one session. I ended up with close to a 50 percent lift. Neither of us can believe it. She had told me at the beginning that I'd never get eighteen-year-old arms. I didn't want teenage arms; I just didn't want them impeding my life. I haven't tried Thermage on any other body part yet, but if my face starts drooping, you can bet that I'm going to have Dr. Copeland zap it.

 Ask the Doctor: *Are new cellulite reducers too good to be true?*

Unfortunately, yes. A lot of people hoped that Vela-Smooth, a device combining infrared, radiofrequency, and massage, would be that much-hoped-for solution. I'm sorry to say that the long-term results haven't been promising. While these modalities can deliver some decrease in skin dimpling, they don't appear to provide a lasting answer to the problem. After investing their time and money in a series of treatments, women often discover several months later that their dreaded cellulite has returned.

I still believe that the future of cellulite minimization is bright; with improved technology, orange peel skin will be conquered, and smooth, even texture will become a reality. We're going to use topical creams, mesotherapy, ultrasound, light energy, and radiofre-

WEIGHT AND SEE

As more men and women use methods such as the gastric band to lose massive quantities of weight, doctors are reporting an increase in patients with tremendous amounts of hanging skin. Currently, one of the main remedies is extensive tissue-tightening surgery, which leaves a very large scar that appears, as I call it, like the mark of Zorro. It's possible to help people avoid that fate by employing a combination of liposuction and radiofrequency. A series of these smaller sessions allows the patient to recover, as well as gives the skin a chance to tighten on its own. This creates minimal scarring while delivering the desired effect.

quency to tackle cellulite. All will help shrink skin and make it look better. Cellulite is an ongoing annoyance, though; new, better therapies will be developed, but they'll still have to be repeated every so often.

ON THE HORIZON

The advances and discoveries in our understanding of disease are beginning to find their way into the skin arena. When we examine the work genetic scientists are doing in cell regulation and modulation and methods for turning off segments of RNA, we can discern the future of skin care. Ideas about redirecting or changing embryonic cells to prevent their maturation introduce a whole new world of thinking about these cells. Stem cell research will also undoubtedly have implications in the way we consider this tissue. In the next ten years, we are going to learn how to reverse the aging process in a healthy manner and arrest negative cellular development.

 Ask the Doctor: *Will you still be performing surgery in twenty years?*

I think I'll be doing less, and I don't believe I'll be doing it in the same fashion. Fewer face-lifts are performed today than a decade ago. Men and women have begun taking care of their skin earlier than people did a generation ago, so their skin holds on to its youthful appearance much longer.

WHAT IT'S ALL ABOUT

The future will bring choice, refinement, and different techniques to regulate skin cells. Eventually, I'm sure that topicals will replace some in-office procedures, such as scar reduction. However, no matter what breakthroughs we accomplish in the lab or in the operating room, you're always going to be at your peak when your skin's foundation is healthy and Creamy. With this book, I hope that I've enabled you to create your best skin possible. I believe in **The Beautiful Skin Workout**, and I believe in you. A vibrant, glowing, fresh face and body are within your grasp. This is your time to take control and make a difference, in a very positive way, of how you look and feel.

Glossary

ablative laser: A skin-resurfacing treatment that removes the entire top layer of skin, exposing the dermis. It is effective at remedying large, hard-to-treat skin defects, but the risk of hyperpigmention and scarring is high.

acne: Includes black- or whiteheads, pimples, cysts, and nodules, which usually occur on the face, neck, chest, back, shoulders, or upper arms as a result of blocked oil glands. While not a severe condition, untreated it can lead to permanent scarring.

alpha hydroxy acid (AHA): A water-soluble chemical exfoliant or superficial peel derived from natural sources such as fruit. AHA helps skin shed superficial cells, creating smoother surface.

alpha-lipoic acid: An antioxidant found in small amounts in liver, broccoli, and potatoes. It deactivates free radicals and helps antioxidant vitamins C and E work to their full potential.

antioxidant: Any of a number of chemicals that reduce oxidative stress. Antioxidants neutralize skin fiber–destroying free radicals.

arbutin: Helps inhibit pigment formation. It is found in the leaves of cranberry and blueberry shrubs and many types of pears, as well as other plants.

argeriline: An amino-peptide that temporarily limits production of neurotransmitters controlling muscle contractions, which relaxes the appearance of wrinkles.

azelaic acid: A topical that works by killing pore-infecting bacteria; often used to treat rosacea and acne.

beta-carotene: An antioxidant found in fruits and vegetables such as mangoes, sweet potatoes, and carrots. It may also lower the risk of cancer and other disease.

beta hydroxy acid: A lipid-soluble chemical exfoliant often used to treat oily skin, due to its ability to penetrate pores and dissolve sebum.

Botox (botulinum toxin type A): The most commonly used form of a bacteria-derived, naturally occurring chemical that, when injected into a muscle, temporarily paralyzes it. This erases wrinkles caused by muscle use. Botox can also be injected to reduce perspiration and headaches. The effects often take a few days to appear.

calcium hydroxylapatite: A viscous filler (marketed as Radiesse) injected to plump deep wrinkles or shape the nose. It can remain in place as long as two years.

carnitine (ergothioneine and thiotaine): An antioxidant found in mushrooms. It helps brighten the skin.

chemical peel: A solution formulated with acids, such as trichloric or glycolic, for the face or body, which removes unwanted tissue layers and promotes regrowth of new, smoother skin.

coenzyme Q10 (idebenone): A fat-soluble antioxidant naturally present in every human cell.

collagen: A strong, fibrous protein inherent in skin. It can be injected into wrinkles and lines to plump them temporarily.

cystic acne: A closed, inflamed pustule that forms underneath the skin's surface due to blocked sebaceous gland; often located at a deeper level than a traditional blemish.

dermis: The layer of skin tissue beneath epidermis. It contains nerve endings, hair follicles, sweat and sebaceous glands, and blood vessels.

DMAE (Dimethylamino ethanol): A hormone produced by the adrenal glands. Applied topically, it helps relax nerves in the skin, giving a relaxed appearance.

elastin: A protein in connective tissue that allows the skin to stretch and resume shape after being contracted.

endovenous laser treatment (EVLT): Employs a laser fiber to destroy larger blood vessels, such as varicose veins, with thermal energy. EVLT is less invasive than surgery and with a shorter recovery period.

epidermis: The outer layer of skin, primarily composed of flat, scalelike cells. The epidermis does not contain blood vessels. As the body produces new dermal cells, older cells in the dermis rise toward the body's surface to form the epidermis.

exfoliate: To remove the surface layer of skin cells, either by chemical or physical means. It encourages cellular turnover, which increases production of collagen.

ferulic acid: An antioxidant found in the seeds and leaves of many plants. It helps antioxidant vitamins C and E to function more efficiently.

fractional skin resurfacing: A procedure involving a fractionated laser, such as Fraxel, ActiveFX, and Lux 1540, which creates tiny pinpricks in the skin's surface, stimulating collagen production underneath. Mild flaking can occur; generally requires fewer sessions than nonablative devices to produce results.

free radical: A highly reactive, unstable molecule missing an electron. To neutralize itself, it often picks electrons off skin cells, weakening them and leading to tissue breakdown.

GABA (gamma-aminobutyric acid): The most widespread inhibitory neurotransmitter in the brain; it prevents natural muscle contraction. Applied to the skin, GABA can help release tissue creases and other fine lines.

glycolic acid: A fruit acid frequently used in chemical peels. It is also employed as a rejuvenating ingredient in skin-care products.

grape seed extract (resveratrol): A potent anti-inflammatory and antioxidant found primarily in the skin of red grapes and also in the seeds.

hyaluronic acid: Water-retaining connective fibers naturally present in the skin. It also is available in an injectable form (under the names Restylane, Hylaform, and Juvaderm), derived either from rooster comb or bacteria, and used to fill wrinkles in the face. It typically remains in tissue up to six months.

hydroquinone: A type of chemical used to break up excess pigment in the skin.

hyperpigmentation: Excessive discoloration of the skin, often caused by sun exposure.

hypopigmentation: White patches on the skin indicating a complete lack of color in tissue, usually the outcome of a botched chemical peel or laser treatment.

infrared: A wavelength of light that penetrates lower levels of skin tissue than do nonablative or fractional resurfacing lasers. It encourages skin tightening and lifting and is noninvasive. Titan is best-known device.

intense pulsed light (IPL): A treatment using multiple light wavelengths to trigger collagen growth and resolve pigmentation issues, such as rosacea and age spots. Gentle and non-specifically directed, IPL may require multiple sessions to produce results.

isoflavone: An estrogenlike hormone found in soybeans. It has antioxidant capabilities and helps reverse the skin thinning that happens with age.

keloid: Red, fibrous scar tissue that forms at the site due to an overproduction of collagen.

kojic acid: An antioxidant found in mushrooms. It helps block pigment synthesis.

lactic acid (mandelic): A form of alpha hydroxy acid derived from milk. It is less irritating than glycolic acid and thus considered a good exfoliating agent for sensitive skin.

light-emitting diodes (LEDs): An extremely low dose of light energy that encourages collagen growth. LEDs may also reduce redness and inflammation following laser treatment.

lutein: An antioxidant available in green, leafy vegetables. It is especially beneficial for the eyes.

lycopene: An antioxidant naturally present in red tomatoes.

melanin: A pigment produced by the body that gives skin a darkened tone and can help protect against ultraviolet rays.

mesotherapy: A treatment in which small, short needles place medications in the juncture between the epidermis and dermis. It can improve lymphatic drainage and the appearance of cellulite.

microdermabrasion: A physical exfoliation technique in which fine crystals are sprayed at the skin, removing the uppermost layer of cells and producing smoother skin. The same crystals may also be added to skin creams for at-home polishing. Either form is effective at reducing fine lines, large pores, and adult acne.

milk thistle (silymarin): An anti-inflammatory and antioxidant. Silymarin is extracted from the plant's seeds and is believed to be the biologically active component.

nonablative laser: Stimulates collagen growth and smooths wrinkles, while leaving the surface of the skin untouched. It is notable for a lack of side effects, such as redness and swelling. Due to its light touch, it may require multiple courses to produce results.

pentapeptides: An amino-acid group that may help prevent muscle contraction.

peptides: An amino-acid compound that encourages collagen growth by mimicking broken strands of skin tissue, encouraging the body to send in repair fibers.

phyllanthus emblica: A small tree found in India. Its extract helps reduce inflammation and regulate pigment production; it's also rich in vitamin C.

poly-L-lactic acid: A filler (marketed as Sculptra) used in larger sections of facial wasting to stimulate the body's collagen production. Initial treatments must be repeated two to four times over a six-week period. The results generally last up to two years.

radiofrequency: A noninvasive procedure that helps tighten and firm the skin by stimulating collagen formation at a deeper level than does light energy. Improvements are immediate and continue for as long as six months. Widely available as Thermage.

retinoid: A class of chemical compounds related to vitamin A that help regulate cell growth. It is popular for reducing acne and psoriasis.

rosacea: A skin disease characterized by redness, bumps, and thickened texture. It is most common in women between the ages of thirty and sixty and those with fair complexions.

salicylic acid: A chemical exfoliant with anti-inflammatory properties. It helps prevent cell clogging inside hair follicles.

scar: A section of fibrous tissue that replaces normal skin after an injury to the dermis.

sepiwhite: An amino acid chain that helps inhibit melanin production.

sun protection factor (SPF): The measure of effectiveness of sunblock or sunscreen. The number correlates to amount of time skin treated with the product can be exposed to UV light before burning versus uncovered tissue.

vitamin A: A fat-soluble compound available in milk and spinach, among other foods. It helps speed cell turnover, increasing collagen stores.

vitamin C: A highly effective water-soluble antioxidant present in especially large amounts in berries and red peppers.

vitamin E: A powerful fat-soluble antioxidant found in vegetable oils and nuts.

waltheria: The extract from this shrub helps inhibit the enzyme related to melanin creation.

wrinkle: A crease in the skin's surface caused by aging, excessive sun exposure, smoking, dehydration, or a combination of these factors.

zinc: A mineral present in almost every human cell, as well as many foods. It is soothing and can treat acne, rosacea, eczema, and psoriasis.

Index

Index

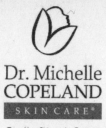

Dr. Michelle COPELAND

SKINCARE®

Trust Your Skin to the Expert.™

We hope you enjoyed *The Beautiful Skin Workout*

Now you too can have great skin by trying our CEAMP Products. Receive 20% off your first purchase!

1. Just log on to www.mcskin.com.
2. Place your order.
3. Enter this special coupon code CEAMPSPECIAL7 at checkout.
4. Offer good until June 31, 2008.

You must be a legal resident of the U.S. or Canada and 18 years or older to be eligible. Void where prohibited.

Any questions, please feel free to call us at 1-866-833-SKIN.
Or go online at www.mcskin.com to check out our full line of products.

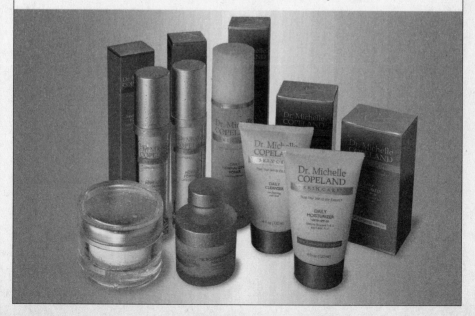